Neuroimaging

edited by
Cristina Marta Del-Ben

Neuroimaging

Edited by Cristina Marta Del-Ben

Republished by InTech

Janeza Trdine 9, 51000 Rijeka, Croatia

Publishing Process Manager Ana Nikolic

Technical Editor Sonja Mujacic

Cover Designer Martina Sirotic

Additional hard copies can be obtained from orders@intechopen.com

Neuroimaging, Edited by Cristina Marta Del-Ben
p. cm.
ISBN 978-953-307-127-5

For EU product safety concerns:
IN TECH d.o.o., Prolaz Marije Krucifikse Kozulić 3, 51000 Rijeka, Croatia,
info@intechopen.com or visit our website at intechopen.com.

Meet the editor

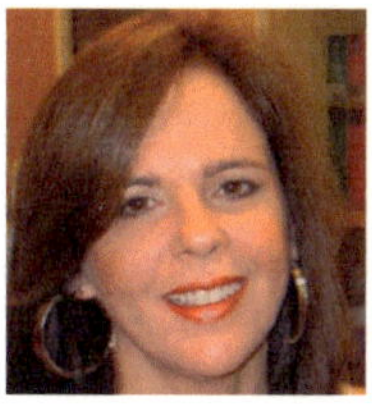

Dr. Del-Ben graduated in Medicine from Londrina State University (1988) and took Medical Residency in Psychiatry (1989 – 1992) at Ribeirão Preto Medical School Clinical Hospital – University of Sao Paulo. She obtained Master's (1995) and Doctoral degree (2000) in Medicine (Mental Health) from University of São Paulo ans took postdoctoral internship at the Psychiatry and Neurosciences Unit of Manchester University, United Kingdom (2002-2003). Coordinated the Mental Health Graduate Program of FMRP-USP (2004-2010). Currently Dr. Del-Ben is an associate professor of the Department of Neurosciences and Behavior from the Faculty of Medicine of Ribeirão Preto of the University of São Paulo and the coordinator of FMRP-USP Medical Residency Program in Psychiatry. She has medical experience with emphasis on Psychiatry, and her main interest in research are Neurobiology of Anxiety and Emotion Processing, Psychiatric Emergencies and Neuroimaging and Diagnosis in Psychiatry.

Contents

Preface

Neuroimaging has become a crucial technique for Neurosciences. Different structural, functional and neurochemical methods, developed in recent decades, have allowed a systematic investigation on the role of neural substrates involved in functions performed by the central nervous system, whether normal or pathological.

Clinical application of neuroimaging specifically for psychological functions or psychiatric disorders is still limited and restricted primarily to the differential diagnosis with other conditions that affect the central nervous system. Nevertheless, the application of neuroimaging techniques has provided a substantial increase in the knowledge regarding the neurobiology of several mental functions. Neuroimaging has been a powerful method to examine the relationship between neurological and psychiatric symptoms, structural and functional changes of the brain, and other biological markers of neurological and psychiatric disorders.

Even though several attempts have been made in order to establish relationships between specific brain abnormalities and specific disorders, an overlap between brain areas and different disorders is still a common finding. Particularly in regard to mental disorders, the results obtained so far suggest that the pathophysiology of these disorders involves dysfunction of integrated circuits or neural networks instead of individual brain regions.

This book includes contributions from the general area of the neuroimaging to the understanding of normal functions and abnormalities of the central nervous system. Chapter 1 presents a critical review of the applications and limits of diffusion imaging techniques and proposes possible solutions to minimize uncertainties related to the area. Chapter 2 gives an insightful review about the principles underlying two different techniques - transcranial magnetic stimulation and functional magnetic resonance imaging - and discusses the possibilities and limitation of the simultaneous application of both. Chapter 3 addresses pharmacological and hormonal modulation of a basic mental function, the emotional faces processing, and its implications for the understanding of anxiety and depression. In chapter 4 the authors give an overview of recent data on the application of positron emission tomography (PET) for the understanding of the molecular basis underlying major depression, a highly prevalent mental disorder, and propose new strategies for the application of PET for further investigations. Chapter 5 discusses neuroimaging data about the neurobiological substrates of drug dependence and also presents studies on vulnerability factors that can predispose individuals to excessive drug intake.

Chapter 6 provides an overview of recent data obtained with spectroscopy, diffusion, perfusion, morphometry and functional neuroimaging techniques about the pathological processes underlying fibromyalgia. Finally, in chapter 7 the authors present new findings obtained by fMRI about the neural substrates involved in the motor recovery of ischemic stroke patients, providing an example of direct application of fMRI in the clinical practice

Editor

Cristina Marta Del-Ben
Division of Psychiatry, Faculty of Medicine of Ribeirão Preto,
University of São Paulo , Brazil

1

On the Reliability of Diffusion Neuroimaging

Jan Klein, Sebastiano Barbieri, Hannes Stuke, Horst K. Hahn
Fraunhofer MEVIS
Germany

Miriam H. A. Bauer, Jan Egger, Christopher Nimsky
Dept. of Neurosurgery, University of Marburg
Germany

1. Introduction

Over the last years, diffusion imaging techniques like DTI, DSI or Q-Ball received increasing attention, especially in the neuroimaging, neurological, and neurosurgical community. An explicit geometrical reconstruction of major white matter tracts has become available by fiber tracking based on diffusion-weighted images. The goal of virtually all fiber tracking algorithms is to compute results which are analogous to what the physicians or radiologists are expecting and an extensive amount of research has therefore been focussed on this reconstruction. However, the results of fiber tracking and quantification algorithms are approximations of the reality due to limited spatial resolution (typically a few millimeters), model assumptions (e.g., diffusion assumed to be Gaussian distributed), user-defined parameter settings, and physical imaging artifacts resulting from diffusion sequences. In this book chapter, we will address the problem of uncertainty in diffusion imaging and we will show possible solutions for minimizing, measuring and visualizing the uncertainty.

The possibility of fiber tracking (FT) and the quantification of diffusion parameters has established an abundance of new clinically useful applications and research studies that focus on neurosurgical planning (Nimsky et al., 2005), monitoring the progression of diseases such as amyotrophic lateral sclerosis (ALS) or multiple sclerosis (MS) (Griffin et al., 2001), establishing surrogate markers used in assessing the grade of brain tumors (Barboriak, 2003), or initiating therapies to ensure the best possible development of children (Pul et al., 2006). Several studies have shown that modified values of fractional anisotropy (FA), relative anisotropy, or diffusion strength (ADC) are indicators of diseases that affect white matter tissue. MS lesions have been investigated by ROI-based analysis and voxel-wise FA comparisons by which FA changes have been shown to occur in areas containing lesions and in areas of normal-appearing white matter. Moreover, methods for tract-based quantification have been developed for which parameters are computed depending on the local curvature or geodesic distance from a user-defined origin. These methods allow to automatically determine DTI-derived parameters along fiber bundles and have already been used to mirror disease progression and executive function in MS (Fink et al., 2009).

Probabilistic methods (Friman et al., 2006) allow for tracking in regions of low anisotropy and are also used to provide a quantitative measure of the probability of the existence of a connection between two regions. These approaches aim at visualizing the uncertainty present in the data by incorporating models of the acquisition process and noise. The uncertainty is assessed by tracking many possible paths originating from a single seed point and by taking the tensor uncertainty into account. Session reproducibility and subject variability of FT algorithms have been examined in (Heiervang et al., 2006). A first comparison of deterministic and probabilistic approaches, both guided solely by the primary eigenvector, in combination with functional localization of brain tumor patients has been given in (Berman et al., 2004).

2. Minimizing, Measuring and Visualizing the Uncertainty in Diffusion Imaging

Correctness, plausibility, and reliability of fiber tracking and quantification techniques have mainly been verified using histologic knowledge (Inglis et al., 1999). In some few animal studies, manganese has already been used as tracer to directly examine the diffusion process (Lin et al., 2001). First quantitative results with respect to precision, uncertainty and reproducibility have also been published (Basser & Pajevic, 2003; Behrens et al., 2003; Jones, 2003). (Behrens et al., 2003) estimate the local probability density using a model describing the diffusion process. The model is used to determine the probability of a connection between two points and, therefore, is used as a quantitative measure for the correctness of the fiber tracking results. (Jones, 2003) makes use of the bootstrapping method in order to compute cones of uncertainties showing a 95% confidence angle. (Basser & Pajevic, 2003) propose a Gaussian distribution that describes the variability of the tensors in the ideal case where the image is only disturbed by radio frequency background noise. In combination with bootstrapping, where the real variability is measured, they are able to benchmark the quality of DTI data. Thereby, wavelet-based methods help them to reduce noise and to preserve borders between different tissue classes.

Phantoms, modeling physically plausible fiber bundles that conform (partially) with human anatomy are important in order to examine different quantification algorithms with respect to the points mentioned above. A phantom must allow to steer the respective DTI data generation under controlled conditions, either using a real MR scanner (*physical phantom*) or by the help of software in a simulation setup (*software phantom*).

Hardware phantoms to assess DTI can be created from physical materials such as silk threads or dialysis tubes (Fieremans, De Deene, Delputte, Ozdemir, Achten & Lemahieu, 2008) and placed in a water basin for acquiring the diffusion weighted images. Hardware phantom experiments for high angular resolution diffusion-weighted imaging (HARDI) data have been proposed recently (Tournier et al., 2008). In (Tournier et al., 2008) three different techniques are compared, namely constrained spherical deconvolution (CSD), super-resolved CSD and Q-ball imaging. It is shown that fiber tracking results, and as a consequence DTI quantification, depend on the employed algorithm's ability to resolve crossing fibers, and to provide accurate estimates of their orientations.

In contrast to hardware phantoms, software phantoms allow for an easy an exact geometrical description of arbitrarily shaped fibers and of an automatic computation of the corresponding diffusion weighted-images so that no MR scanner is needed. (Basser et al., 2002) describe fibers by simple 2D rings in tensor fields, whereas other authors (Gössl et al., 2002) define fibers by cylindric tubes in 3D tensor fields. Thereby, tracts are defined by circular helixes. A mathematical framework for simulating the partial volume between fiber and background tissue has been proposed in (Leemans et al., 2005). The authors obtain a model of a fiber bundle by parameterizing the various features which characterize the bundle. Their results show that a higher correspondence between experimental and synthetic DTI data exists when the modeling a nonconstant fiber density across bundles.

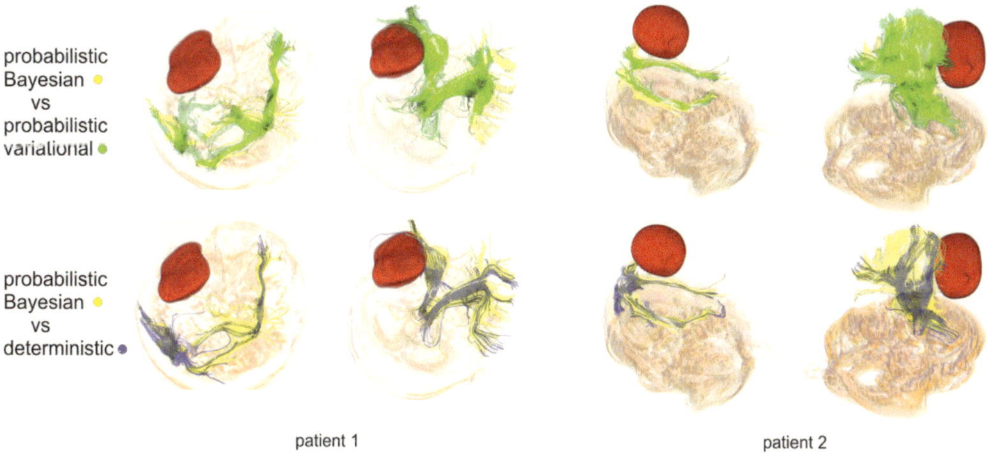

Fig. 1. Qualitative comparisons of fiber tracking for two glioma patients (Klein et al., 2010). We tracked two important structures, the pyramidal tract and the optical tract. Patient 1: frontotemporal glioma (grade 4), patient 2: progressive astrocytoma (grade 2).

In the following sections, we will go into more detail and will give several examples. Section 3 describes how uncertainty due to different tracking algorithms can be visualized and quantified. The next section will illustrate a software phantom for estimating the boundary of tracked fiber bundles. Section 5 summarizes an alternative algorithm for computing a safety hull around the fibers. Finally, we present a new algorithm for visualizing the uncertainty of the reconstruction by the fiber orientation distribution function (fODF), which is a probability distribution on a sphere.

3. Comparing Probabilistic and Deterministic Fiber Tracking

In the following, we will summarize our experiences with comparing probabilistic and deterministic fiber tracking (Klein et al., 2010) and will show which algorithm should be used under which circumstances. For that purpose, we focus on two patient groups: glioma patients and MS patients. Whereas tumors can infiltrate or displace white matter fiber tracts, MS lesions do not necessarily influence the localization or structure of axonal fibers. Rather, the lesions and the corresponding de- and remyelinization may influence the diffusion parameters along the fibers (Fink et al., 2009). Thus, for both groups, we perform FT of bundles of interest, i.e., bundles near the tumor or bundles which can be influenced by lesions. In the case of tumor patients, we mainly focused on qualitative comparisons and visually compared the results in order to assess the differences. Furthermore, we determined the volume of a sheath which wraps the fibers in order to estimate the differences. For the MS patients, we also performed a quantification of several DTI parameters along the tracked bundles.

In the following, we briefly describe the FT algorithms implemented in MeVisLab, our research and development platform (MeVisLab 2.0, 2010) which we used for comparison purpose. Our probabilistic Bayesian approach (Friman et al., 2006) is well-studied and has been used by several other authors, such as (Oguz et al., 2009). Thus, this approach is our first choice for probabilistic FT. The necessary modeling and estimation of fiber orientation and connection can be described at both global and local levels. At the global level, a theoretical foundation for estimating the probability of a connection between two areas in the brain has

been given. At the local level, probability density functions of the fiber orientation can be derived in a theoretically justified way via Bayes' theorem. In addition, a theorem has been integrated that facilitates the estimation of parameters in a constrained version of the popular tensor model of water diffusion.
Although we have fully parallelized the Bayesian approach, its high computation time inhibits use in routine clinical tasks. Thus, we propose another approach for FT similar to bootstrapping methods (Chung et al., 2006; Jones et al., 2005), but which is faster and does not need several repetitions of the diffusion-weighted images. The method, which we have named variational noise FT, allows an efficient computation of diffusion-weighted images with user-defined noise while retaining the MRI noise characteristics. The essential idea is to add complex Gaussian noise to the magnitude images (Hahn et al., 2006) and to track the fibers for each artificially computed diffusion-weighted data set.
For a fair comparison between both probabilistic approaches, the noise of the diffusion-weighted images used for the Bayesian method should match the noise of the images computed by the variational noise technique.
The deterministic FT algorithm which we use (Schlueter et al., 2005) to compare with both probabilistic approaches is based on the deflection-based approach by (Weinstein et al., 1999) and makes use of the full diffusion tensor information during tracking. In contrast, commonly employed streamline-based algorithms, such as the FACT (fiber assignment by continuous tracking) method (Mori et al., 1999), only consider the largest eigenvector representing the main diffusion direction. In comparison to the method described in (Weinstein et al., 1999), we added a moving average estimation of the fiber curvature and anisotropy to the tracking algorithm, which leads to more accurate tracking dynamics and more robust termination criteria.

3.1 Qualitative comparisons of fiber tracking (glioma patients)

For the qualitative analysis, magnetic resonance images of tumor patients were obtained using a 3T scanner (Siemens Trio, Erlangen, Germany). The subjects were supine and a head coil with a circularly polarized array was used with 2D DTI echo planar imaging, 12 diffusion directions and 5 repetitions. The sequence parameters were: repetition time (TR) 6400 msec, echo time (TE) 91 msec, field of view (FOV) 240 mm, voxel size $2.5 \times 2.5 \times 2.5 mm^3$, 50 slices, and scanning time of 8 minutes. Autoshimming and phase correction were activated.
From a large pool of data sets of glioma patients, we selected some patients for a qualitative comparison. All selected patients have progressive gliomas (grade 4) or progressive astrocytomas (grade 2) next to the pyramidal and the optical tracts. To track the pyramidal tracts, seed regions within the capsula interna were chosen, while for tracking the optical tracts, seed regions in the occipital lobe were used. In all cases, exclusion ROIs (regions of interest) were used to discard unwanted fibers. Moreover, we propose to measure the volume of the sheath that encloses the single fiber tracts. To compute the sheath, we propose a neighboring cells algorithm based on the well-known marching cubes algorithm with which a volume (image) is scanned by discretization into cells. The necessary input volume is determined by voxelizing the 3D fiber tracts.
Some of the qualitative results can be found in Fig. 1. In nearly all cases, both probabilistic approaches are superior to the deterministic algorithm. In particular, fibers at the marginal regions of the white matter are more precisely tracked if the probabilistic algorithms are used. Consequently, the sheath volumes differ substantially for the different algorithms (probabilis-

tic results are about 30% higher on average). The differences between the variational noise tracking approach and the Bayesian approach are very small for all patients.

3.2 Quantitative comparisons of fiber tracking (multiple sclerosis patients)

For the quantitative analysis, magnetic resonance images of relapsing-remitting MS patients and healthy controls (10 patients, 10 healthy volunteers) were obtained using a 1.5T scanner (Siemens Avanto, Erlangen, Germany). The subjects were supine and a head coil with a circularly polarized array was used with 2D DTI echo planar imaging, 30 diffusion directions and 2 repetitions. The sequence parameters were: repetition time (TR) 8000 msec, echo time (TE) 100 msec, field of view (FOV) 230 mm, voxel size $2.0 \times 2.0 \times 2.7mm^3$, 55 slices, and a scanning time of 8 minutes. Autoshimming and phase correction were activated.

We have tested both the deterministic and the probabilistic FT (Bayesian) to determine whether and how they allow the detection of differences of diffusion-derived parameters between relapsing-remitting MS patients and healthy controls (10 patients, 10 healthy volunteers). For that purpose, we decided to quantify the superior longitudinal fasciculus (SLF) which has already been shown to be a structure for which differences between MS patients and healthy volunteers can be determined very well using deterministic FT (Fink et al., 2009). After extracting the right and left SLF, diffusion-derived parameters such as the FA, axial diffusivity, radial diffusivity, and diffusion strength were obtained along the tracts, and average values were computed. Then these values were recoded linearly to better permit statistical examination. For extracting the SLFs, only fiber tracts were considered which were included by two crop ROIs and values were only computed between those two crop ROIs. More precisely, each fiber is resampled so that all fibers consist of n equidistantly distributed fiber points. Using the resampled fibers, an average center line is computed, used to determine n reference planes depending on the local curvature of the center line. Afterwards, a reference plane is used to determine an average diffusion value at a certain position of the bundle by considering one diffusion value per fiber with the nearest distance to that plane.

The number of fibers of the probabilistic tracking has been aligned with the number of fibers of the deterministic tracking. This process occurs before the tracked structure has been cropped to the focus of interest in the SLF to ensure a valid comparison of the parameters after cropping. Furthermore, common parameters such as minimal FA must be adjusted for both algorithms.

The quantitative results can be found in Tab. 1 and Tab. 2. In two of the MS cases, fiber tracts could not be determined between both crop ROIs by the deterministic approach. Thus, these two cases were discarded. We used analysis of variance (ANOVA) through GLM (general linear model) for repeated measurements to analyze the sensitivity of the deterministic and the probabilistic method for pathological alterations in the MS patients. The FA and ADC values of the SLF left and the SLF right were used as dependent variables. The patient versus healthy control status is used as independent variable (between-subject factor), the hemisphere and the type of algorithm (deterministic/probabilistic) as within-subject factors. For the ADC values, there is a main effect for the cerebral hemisphere [F(1,16): 11.027, $p < 0.01$], a main effect for the algorithm used (deterministic vs. probabilistic) [F(1,16): 4.444, $p = 0.05$] and a significant interaction between algorithm used and patient groups [F(1,16): 4.444, p = 0.05]. Moreover, the independent group factor is also significant [F(1,17): 12.085, $p < 0.01$].

Patients had higher ADC values than healthy controls (3.625 vs. 2.25), right hemisphere ADC values are higher than left hemisphere ADC values (3.194 vs. 2.681), in healthy controls the ADC values did not differ between deterministic and probabilistic algorithm (2.25 vs. 2.25),

but in patients the probabilistic model yielded higher values than the deterministic algorithm (3.75 vs. 3.5). Note that these values are not the empiric data itself, but estimated marginal means, thus error-corrected values based on our empiric data.
For the FA values, the only significant effect is a main effect for the cerebral hemisphere [F(1,16): 5.47, p = 0.03].
The number of fibers after the cropping varies widely not only between different persons, but also between hemispheres of the same brain. Statistics show that the probabilistic algorithm tracks an average of 254 fibers (SD=199), whereas the deterministic algorithm tracks an average of 188 fibers (SD=167). The standard deviation is high, that it seems impossible to interpret these results at first glance. However, the correlation between the probabilistically and deterministically gained numbers of fibers, found by Pearson test to be 0.89, shows that the trend between the algorithms is congruent. This indicates that the variance of the number of fibers is not due to the type of algorithm or chance, but primarily due to the underlying image data. Additionally, this highly variant but congruent trend indicates a high sensibility towards inter-individual differences in image data and demonstrates reliable algorithms.

	FA (prob.)	**FA (det.)**	**ADC (prob.)**	**ADC (det.)**
mean (right)	0.4130	0.4120	0.000716	0.000717
stddev (right)	0.0285	0.0311	$2.84 \cdot 10^{-5}$	$2.58 \cdot 10^{-5}$
mean (left)	0.4190	0.4170	0.000692	0.000692
stddev (left)	0.0300	0.0352	$2.89 \cdot 10^{-5}$	$2.69 \cdot 10^{-5}$

Table 1. Control group. FA: fractional anisotropy, ADC: diffusion strength.

	FA (prob.)	**FA (det.)**	**ADC (prob.)**	**ADC (det.)**
mean (right)	0.3680	0.3740	0.000810	0.000809
stddev (right)	0.0405	0.0390	$7.36 \cdot 10^{-5}$	$7.74 \cdot 10^{-5}$
mean (left)	0.3900	0.3910	0.000771	0.000767
stddev (left)	0.0403	0.0416	$7.53 \cdot 10^{-5}$	$7.33 \cdot 10^{-5}$

Table 2. MS patients. FA: fractional anisotropy, ADC: diffusion strength.

3.3 Discussion

Our qualitative results have shown that both probabilistic approaches are superior for tracking fibers near tumors or MS lesions with respect to completeness, quality and coverage of anatomical structures at their borders. Under the condition that all approaches are parameterized so that they track the same initial number of fibers, the probabilistic approaches are able to compute more fibers that pass two distant crop ROIs, indicating that fewer fibers were aborted during the fiber tracking process. The variational noise fiber tracking produces qualitatively very similar results compared to the Bayesian approach, but is computationally less expensive, thus, enhancing its appeal for clinical applications.
The quantitative results in combination with the qualitative results have shown that the probabilistic fiber tracking is more sensitive than the deterministic approach, especially if measuring the ADC values. The statistically significant interaction effect for ADC values between the

algorithm used (probabilistic/deterministic) and the health status results from the fact that on one level of the between-subjects factor (healthy volunteers) the algorithm used has no influence on the ADC scores, on the other level (patients) it influences the values. One can interpret this effect as a brain anatomy related effect of the algorithms used to generate the ADC values. The normal or more ideal brain anatomy of healthy volunteers allows less differentiation between the methods than does the pathological brain anatomy of patients. For quantification, we concentrated on one important fiber structure, the SLF, however, samples of other structures have shown similar results.

It is advisable to combine the quantitative and qualitative results to obtain an overall picture. For example, some MS patients could not be added to the quantitative analysis because only the probabilistic algorithm is able to produce processable results. This indicates that in clinical cases with brain lesions or neuronal diseases, the probabilistic algorithm is the method of choice. Although first papers have already proposed to implement probabilistic approaches on the GPU (McGraw & Nadar, 2007), this field of research should be examined in the future as probabilistic approaches are still an order of magnitude slower than deterministic solutions.

4. Assessing Fiber Tracking Accuracy via Diffusion Tensor Software Models

One of the major hurdles when developing fiber tracking algorithms is that hardware or software models of fiber bundles are needed in order to asses their validity and precision. It is therefore necessary to develop phantoms with a known fiber network. Software models have the advantage that they can be easily modified to account for different scanner parameters, image noise or artifacts. While much of the previous work has focused on simple phantoms in which fiber bundles were represented as cylindrical tubes or helices (see for example (Fieremans, De Deene, Delputte, Ozdemir, D'Asseler, Vlassenbroeck, Deblaere, Achten & Lemahieu, 2008; Gössl et al., 2002; Lori et al., 2002)), in this section we suggest a framework in which it is possible to realistically model specific neural fiber bundles, simulating both the smooth transition between the actual white matter pathway and the surrounding tissue and the partial volume effects caused by the possible contemporary presence of white matter, grey matter and cerebrospinal fluid in one voxel.

We focus on generating a phantom of the corticospinal tract. Afterwards, we reconstruct the modeled tract by means of a fiber tracking algorithm and make a quantitative analysis of the algorithm's accuracy. This information is used to estimate what an appropriate safety margin around the tracked fibers should be and to analyze after which length the first fibers start to leave the modeled fiber bundle. Lastly, we suggest an efficient algorithm to construct safety hulls around the tracked fibers.

4.1 DTI Model Framework

In this section, we start by introducing the general framework that we use to generate the diffusion tensor model. Next, we provide details on how we model different tissues and white matter pathways. After an accuracy analysis of the employed fiber tracking algorithm, we conclude by suggesting an algorithm to construct safety hulls around the tracked fibers.

In order to generate a synthetic tensor field, we start by computing a set a of diffusion-weighted (DW) images (one image for each corresponding gradient direction). The diffusion-weighted signal is modeled according to the CHARMED model proposed in (Assaf & Basser, 2005; Assaf et al., 2004). This model contains a hindered extra-axonal compartment as well as a restricted intra-axonal compartment. We restrict ourselves to the hindered model, which

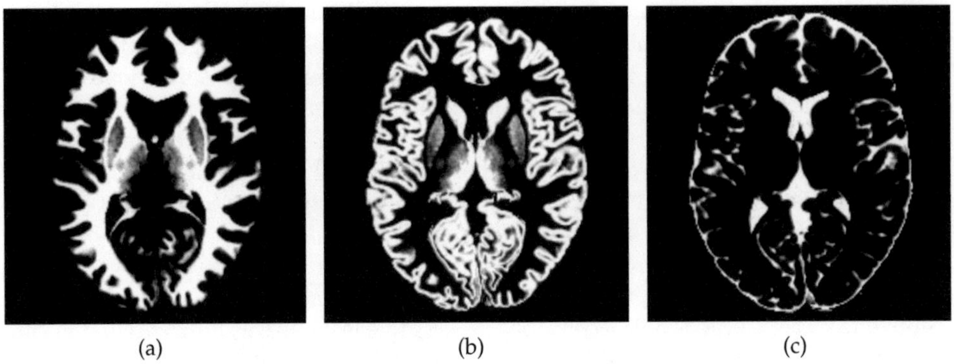

Fig. 2. (a): An example slice of the white matter volume. (b): The grey matter volume. (c): The cerebrospinal fluid volume.

gives rise to an effective diffusion tensor and primarily explains the Gaussian signal attenuation observed at low b values. Let us denote the diffusion time by Δ and set

$$\mathbf{q} = \frac{\gamma \mathbf{g} \delta}{2\pi}$$

Here γ is the proton gyromagnetic ratio, $\mathbf{g}$ is the vector whose magnitude is the strength of the applied diffusion gradient and whose direction is along the axis of the applied diffusion gradient, δ is the width of the diffusion pulse gradient. In this case, the net signal attenuation is given by

$$E(\mathbf{q}, \Delta) = \sum_{i=1}^{M} f_h^i \cdot E_h^i(\mathbf{q}, \Delta) \tag{1}$$

where the f_h^i are the T_2 weighted volume fractions of the hindered compartments, $E_h^i(\mathbf{q}, \Delta)$ is the normalized MR echo signal from the i-th hindered compartment in a voxel. The CHARMED model assumes a cylindrically symmetric tensor model ($\lambda_1 \neq \lambda_2 = \lambda_3$) and denotes the diffusion coefficients parallel and perpendicular to the axon's fiber by $\lambda_{\|}$ and $\lambda_{\perp}$ respectively. In similar manner, q may be written as $\mathbf{q} = \mathbf{q}_{\|} + \mathbf{q}_{\perp}$. For details on the computation of $\mathbf{q}_{\|}$ and $\mathbf{q}_{\perp}$ see (Assaf et al., 2004). Then $E_h^i(\mathbf{q}, \Delta)$ is given by

$$E_h^i(\mathbf{q}, \Delta) = e^{-4\pi^2(\Delta-(\delta/3))|q_{\|}|^2\lambda_{\|}} + e^{-4\pi^2(\Delta-(\delta/3))|q_{\perp}|^2\lambda_{\perp}}$$

It is known that noise in magnitude magnetic resonance data is Rician distributed (Gudbjartsson & Patz, 1995). As suggested in (Hahn et al., 2006), such noise distribution may be simulated in the image by computing $|E(\mathbf{q}, \Delta) + \tilde{N}(0, \sigma^2)|$, where $\tilde{N}(0, \sigma^2)$ is a Gaussian distributed complex variable with mean 0 and variance σ^2. Using standard fitting procedures, we use the DW images to compute the tensor valued image.

4.2 A Model based on Simulated Brain Data

Given the framework presented in Section 4.1, we need to specify the fractions of tissue present in each voxel with the corresponding T_2 and diffusion properties. To this end, we build upon the BrainWeb project at McGill University (Bra, n.d.; Collins et al., 1998). The

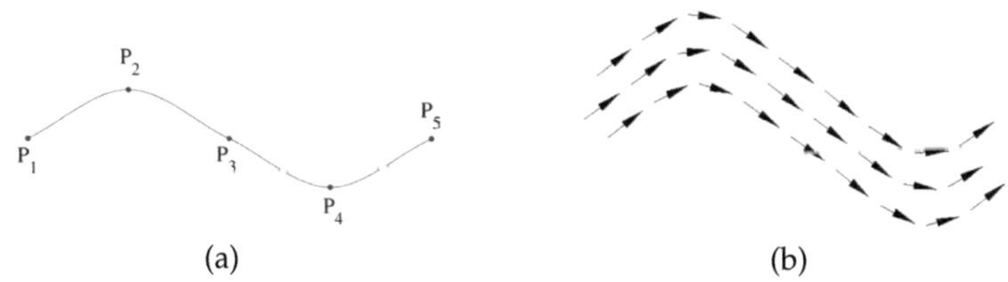

Fig. 3. (a): Example curve interpolating the control points $\{P_i\}$ and forming the backbone of the modeled fiber bundle. (b): Schematic representation of the main diffusion directions of the tensors within the modeled fiber bundle.

BrainWeb project provides a dataset created by means of 27 low-noise scans (T_1 weighted gradient echo acquisitions with TR/TE/FA $= 18\text{ms}/10\text{ms}/30°$) of the same individual, coregistered in stereotaxic space where they were subsampled and intensity averaged (Holmes et al., 1998). By means of a modified minimum-distance classifier, ten volumetric datasets that define the spatial distribution for different tissues were created. In these images, the voxel intensity is proportional to the fraction of tissue within the voxel. In our model we make use of the white matter, grey matter and cerebrospinal fluid volumes, an example slice of each volume is shown in Fig. 2. The volumes are defined at a 1mm isotropic voxel grid, with dimensions $181 \times 217 \times 181$ (XxYxZ). Other tissue volumes that might be included in our model in later work include fat, skin, glial matter, and connective tissue.
To each fraction of tissue in a voxel we assign a main diffusion direction and the eigenvalues of the cylindrically symmetric diffusion tensor. The resulting signal attenuation is then computed according to Equation 1. For the above tissues, the average eigenvalues of the diffusion tensors have been measured and reported in (Bhagat & Beaulieu, 2004; Partridge et al., 2004; Pierpaoli et al., 1996), from which we derive the eigenvalues for our model written in Table 3. In case we do not model one or more white matter tracts to go through a voxel V, we assign a

	T_2 (ms)	$\lambda_{\parallel}$ (10^{-4}mm^2/s)	$\lambda_{\perp}$ (10^{-4}mm^2/s)
White Matter	70	11.30±0.7	5.15±0.3
Grey Matter	83	9.90±0.4	7.05±0.3
Cerebrospinal Fluid	329	36.00±2.3	30.36±1.8

Table 3. T_2 values and tensor eigenvalues used in the BrainWeb-based model for the different tissues.

random main diffusion direction to each tissue portion present in V. However, we let the main diffusion directions corresponding to a given tissue type vary smoothly in space, in order to have, at least locally, a realistic change in tensor orientation.
Otherwise, if V has a white matter tissue portion and there are one or more fiber bundles going through it, the main diffusion direction depends on these bundles. Details on the modeling of fiber bundles and on setting the main diffusion direction are given in the following Section 4.3.

4.3 Modeling White Matter Pathways

In order to model a white matter pathway we start by defining a tuple of n control points $\{P_i\}_{i=1,\ldots,n}$ in $\mathbb{R}^3$ through which the fiber bundle should go. To obtain a smooth backbone of a fiber bundle from just a few control points, we perform cubic spline interpolation on $\{P_i\}$. For simplicity we choose Catmull-Rom splines, which are defined by two points P_i, P_{i+1} and two tangent vectors T_i, T_{i+1}. The tangent vectors are computed by

$$T_j = \frac{1}{2} \cdot (T_{j+1} - T_{j-1})$$

Then the evolution of the parametric curve $s_i(t) = (x_i(t), y_i(t), z_i(t))^T$ with $t \in [0,1]$ and connecting P_i and P_{i+1} is given for example in x-dimension by

$$x_i(t) = \begin{pmatrix} t^3 & t^2 & t & 1 \end{pmatrix} \cdot \begin{pmatrix} 2 & -2 & 1 & 1 \\ -3 & 3 & -2 & -1 \\ 0 & 0 & 1 & 0 \\ 1 & 0 & 0 & 0 \end{pmatrix} \cdot \begin{pmatrix} P_{i_x} \\ P_{i+1_x} \\ T_{i_x} \\ T_{i+1_x} \end{pmatrix}$$

and similarly in the other dimensions. Concatenating the different splines $\{s_i\}$ we have a differential 3D curve s connecting P_1 to P_n. See Fig. 3(a) for an example curve.
Next, we resample the spline s at (small) equidistant t steps and obtain a final set of points which we denote by $\{r_i\}_{i=1,\dots,N}$. As suggested in (Leemans et al., 2005), we define a piecewise differential 3D space curve $t(r)$, which is 1 if r is on the backbone of the fiber and 0 else. $t(r)$ is given by

$$t(r) = \sum_{i=1}^{N-1} \int_0^1 \delta[r - (r_i + \alpha\Delta_i)] \mathrm{d}\alpha$$

where δ denotes the Dirac-delta distribution and α is a parametrization variable. To model the non-constant fiber density we convolve the fiber trajectory $t(r)$ with a kernel $k(r)$:

$$T(r) = t(r) * k(r) = \sum_{i=1}^{N-1} \underbrace{\int_0^1 k[r - (r_i + \alpha\Delta_i)] \mathrm{d}\alpha}_{\equiv T^i(r)}$$

Specifically we choose the saturated kernel

$$k(r) = \frac{\operatorname{erf}\left(\frac{w+2\|r\|}{2\sqrt{2}\sigma}\right) + \operatorname{erf}\left(\frac{w-2\|r\|}{2\sqrt{2}\sigma}\right)}{2\operatorname{erf}\left(\frac{w}{2\sqrt{2}\sigma}\right)}$$

where erf is the error function, the parameter w controls the width of the fiber bundle and σ controls the variance of the Gaussian decay.
We set the percentage $P(r)$ of white matter occupied by the fiber in the voxel at r by

$$P(r) = \frac{T(r)}{\max_{r \in \mathbb{R}^3} T(r)}$$

The remaining white matter is modeled as having a random direction. In case there are several fibers which contribute to a voxel, we generally proceed as above, with the difference that we may have to rescale each contribution by the sum of all contributions, so that the latter sum is less or equal to one (100%).

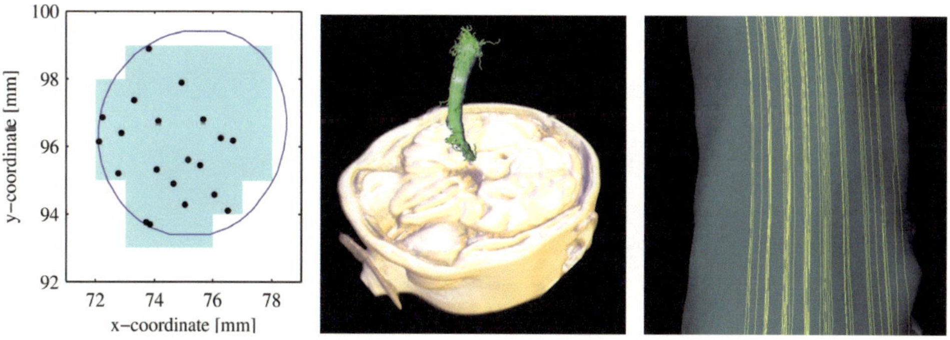

(a) (b) (c)

Fig. 4. (a): Cross section of the modeled corticospinal tract. The location of the tracked fibers is shown as dots. The voxels recognized by the safety-hull algorithm as part of the fiber bundle are overlayed in light blue. The parameters were $T_{\text{dist}}=4\text{mm}$, $T_{\text{FA}}=0.1$, $T_{\text{BD}}=0.07$, $T_{\text{angle}}=3°$. (b): Safety hull rendered with the tracked fibers. (c): Detail of the computed safety hull, showing its asymmetry with respect to the tracked fibers.

The main diffusion direction e_1 of a fiber at r is computed as a weighted sum of the vector lines Δ_i:

$$e_1(r) = \frac{\sum_{i=1}^{N-1} T^i(r)\Delta_i}{\left\|\sum_{i=1}^{N-1} T^i(r)\Delta_i\right\|}$$

A schematic representation of the main diffusion directions of the tensors is given in Fig. 3(b).

4.4 Fiber Tracking Analysis

With the help of a physician having experience with DTI, we define the backbone of the right corticospinal tract. It is initially defined by 18 points and the parameters for the convolution kernel are w=12mm and σ=0.5. After resampling it consists of 968 points at a distance of 0.1mm. It is important to note that the thickness of a fiber bundle does not only depend on the kernel width, but also on the actual presence of white matter in the different voxels. After the fiber has been added to the model, we track it using the advection-diffusion based fiber tracking algorithm presented in (Schlueter et al., 2005), see also Section 3. In our implementation, the resulting tracked fibers are represented by several linearly connected points. To evaluate our algorithm, we compute the Hausdorff distance between one point of the spline-interpolated fiber backbone and the points of the tracked fibers. Given that the fibers are sampled densely enough, this distance provides a good approximation of the maximal distance between the fibers in the model and those that are tracked.

4.5 An Algorithm to Compute Safety Hulls

In the previous sections we have suggested a way to generate DT software models of specific neural fiber bundles and to analyze the error of the tracked fibers. We are now going to suggest an efficient algorithm to better estimate the extent of a tracked fiber bundle. The resulting data will be visualized my means of hulls around the tracked fibers, which we will denote by "safety hulls". We test our algorithm both on the BrainWeb-based phantom and on the real magnetic resonance scans of a patient. The suggested algorithm to compute safety

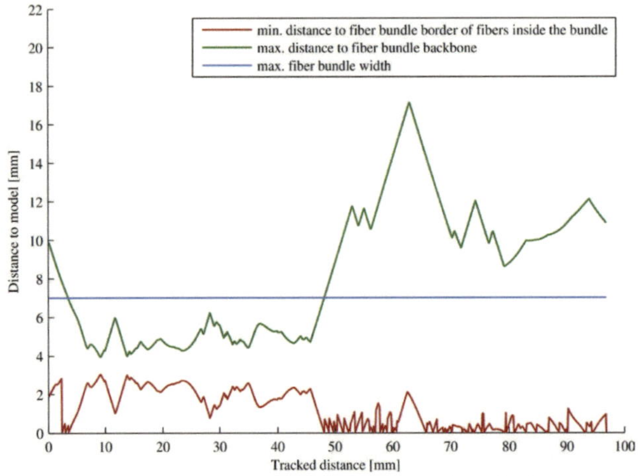

Fig. 5. Maximum distance between tracked fibers and modeled fiber bundle backbone.

hulls basically relies on dilating the tracked fibers if several threshold conditions are met. The algorithm proceeds as follows:

- Sample the tracked fibers and mark the image-voxels in which the sampled points lie. We will denote this set of voxels by $\{V_i\}$.
- For each voxel $V \in \{V_i\}$ search in a $n \times n \times n$ box centered at V. Out of this search box, mark a voxel $\tilde{V}$ if it satisfies the following threshold conditions:
  - The distance between V and $\tilde{V}$ should be smaller than T_{dist}.
  - The difference in FA between V and $\tilde{V}$ should be smaller than T_{FA}.
  - The difference in bulk diffusivity (BD) between V and $\tilde{V}$ should be smaller than T_{BD}.
  - The angle between the main diffusion directions of V and $\tilde{V}$ should be smaller than T_{angle}.

  We will denote the resulting larger set of Voxels by $\{\tilde{V}\}_j$.
- Denoising step: do a connected-component analysis on $\{\tilde{V}\}_j$ and discard groups of voxels smaller than a predefined volume .
- For visualization purposes, fit a smooth surface to the resulting voxel set, giving the desired safety hulls.

In our inclusion criterion, the BD threshold is mainly used to differentiate between cerebrospinal fluid, tumor tissue, and regions of white or grey matter. On the other hand, FA has been shown to be highly heterogeneous in normal brain parenchyma and may be used as a criterion to differentiate between different white matter tracts. For measurements of tensor eigenvalues in the different brain regions and a detailed analysis we refer to (Bhagat & Beaulieu, 2004; Partridge et al., 2004; Pierpaoli et al., 1996). As far as the connected-component analysis step of the algorithm is concerned, we make use of 6-connectivity in 3D and discard groups of voxels with a volume smaller than 50ml.

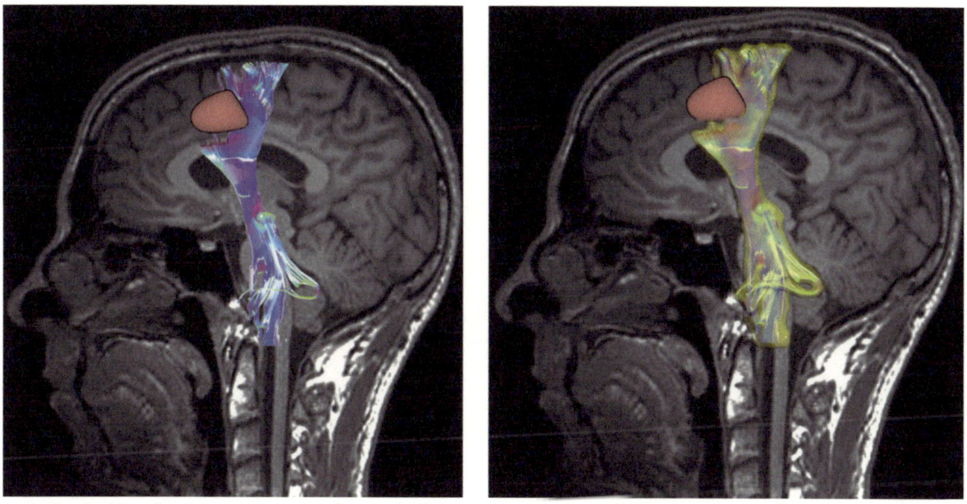

Fig. 6. Left: Tracked corticospinal tract of a tumor patient. The segmented tumor is shown in red. Right: Example visualization how margin around fibers can be visualized.

4.6 Results

The remaining parameters used to compute the diffusion weighted images according to Equation 1 are reported in Table 4. We select a region at the level of the internal capsule to start

	Default value
voxel size	$1 \times 1 \times 1$ mm^3
number of gradients	6
gradient strength	20 T/m
diffusion time	40 msec
pulse width	35 msec
gyromagnetic ratio	$2.675 \cdot 10^8$ rad/sT
thermal noise variance	100
fiber tracking step length	1 mm

Table 4. Parameters used to compute the signal attenuation.

the tracking of the corticospinal tract. After the tracking, fibers which are obviously not part of the corticospinal tract are excluded from the result. Fig. 5 shows the tracked fibers and the distance plot. More in detail, the plot shows on one hand the maximum distance between fiber backbone and tracked fibers, on the other the minimum distance between fibers correctly tracked inside the bundle and the border of the bundle model (note that in the midbrain the latter distance may also be constrained by the actual presence of white matter).

We observe that fibers are tracked correctly inside the modeled fiber bundle between 3.5 and 48mm. Given that the fiber tracking seed was close to 25mm, this indicates that after a distance of approximately 20mm the first fibers leave the modeled bundle. When fibers are tracked correctly inside the bundle, the maximum distance to the fiber bundle border varies between 2 and 3mm, which this experiment indicates to be an appropriate safety margin. We start by

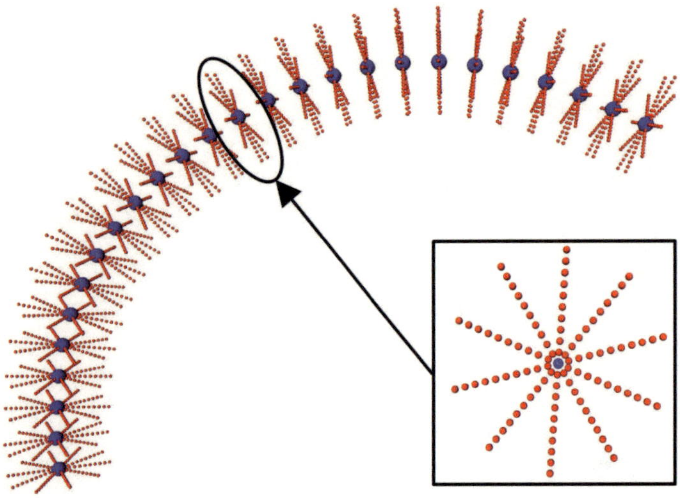

Fig. 7. The graph-based approach for estimating the boundary of fiber bundles, shown in Section 5, determines evaluation points around the calculated centerline of the bundle.

testing the safety hull generating algorithm on the tracked corticospinal tract from Section 4.2. The resulting hull is shown in Fig. 4. Particularly, from Fig. 4(c) we notice the asymmetry of the safety hull with respect to the tracked fibers. Finally, we test the algorithm on a real magnetic resonance dataset of a tumor patient (diffusion weighted images with TR/TE/FA= 6400ms/91ms/90°, voxel size is 2.5mm isotropic). The runtime of the algorithm was a few seconds on a QuadCore personal computer. Fig. 6 shows an example visualization how the safety hulls could be visualized.

4.7 Discussion

In this section, we have described the creation of realistic DTI software models. These can be used as ground truth to test various fiber tracking algorithms. A first quantitative analysis of the advection-diffusion based fiber tracking algorithm suggests that, in the considered experiment, the first fibers leave the modeled bundle after approximately 20mm and that a safety margin of 2-3mm seems appropriate. Future work includes analyzing the precision of the algorithm in the presence of kissing or crossing fibers. We would also like to systematically analyze how precision varies in relation with the underlying image data (testing different values for image noise or artifacts, thickness of the fiber bundle, fractional anisotropy of the tensors) or in relation with fiber tracking parameters (such as step length, density of seed points). Moreover, fiber tracking results should be compared with those of other approaches, such as for example probabilistic ones. In the following Section 4.5, we suggested an algorithm to estimate the extent of a fiber bundle based on the tracked fibers and the underlying image data. The algorithm basically relies on dilating the tracked fibers if threshold conditions on voxel distance, FA, BD, and main diffusion direction difference are met. Results are visualized as semi-transparent hulls around the tracked fibers. The algorithm was tested both on one of our DTI phantoms and on a real magnetic resonance dataset. As with every parameter-dependent algorithm, the question of the optimal set of parameters arises, which shall be dealt with in the future. Ultimately, this work should help clinicians in better understanding the precision of generated fiber tracking results.

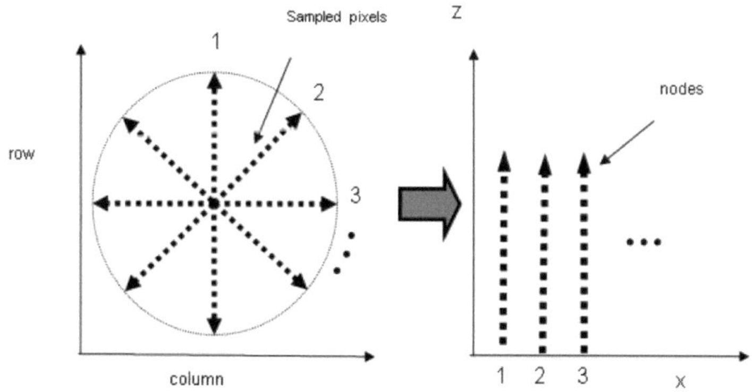

Fig. 8. Graph construction by unfolding of planes.

5. A Graph-based Approach for Boundary Estimation

Besides fiber tracking there are other approaches for fiber bundle segmentation and boundary estimation like volume growing (Merhof et al., 2005) or a graph-based min-cut segmentation depending on fractional anisotropy maps that will be discussed in the following section.

The segmentation starts with the choice of the fiber bundle for segmentation described by two manually placed regions of interest (ROIs) as start and end of the segmentation result. With the help of deflection based fiber tracking only tracked fibers within both ROIs are kept and cropped at the ROIs. Based on the resulting fibers a centerline of the fiber bundle is calculated like described by (Klein et al., 2007).

After the centerline calculation a set of evaluation points is created in the centerline's surrounding like shown in Fig. 7.

Therefore, the centerline is sampled at n points p_i, $i \in [1..n]$. For each of these point a plane upright to the local centerlines direction, given by $p_{i+1} - p_i$ for $i \in [1..n-1]$ and $p_n - p_{n-1}$ for $i = n$, is calculated. Within each of these planes l rays are sent out radially. Each ray is then sampled at m points with distance d between each of them. Each of this points is labeled with $v_{i,j,k}$ where $i \in [1..n]$ describes the plane, $j \in [1..l]$ describes the ray within the plane and $k \in [1..m]$ describes the evaluation point along the ray within the plane.

For the construction of the directed graph $G = (V, E)$ the sampled planes are now unfolded in clockwise direction beginning with the ray at 12 o'clock like shown in Fig. 8 according to (Egger et al., 2009; 2008; Li et al., 2004a;b; 2006; Wu & Chen, 2002).

The set of nodes consists of all evaluation points $v_{i,j,k}$ ($i \in [1..n], j \in [1..l], k \in [1..m]$) and two additional nodes v_{sink} and v_{source}. The construction of weighted edges consists of different steps and is partly based on a cost function $c(v_{i,j,k})$ for every node $v_{i,j,k}$. The used scalar cost function $c(v_{i,j,k})$ is derived from the scalar fractional anisotropy maps of the underlying tensor data:

1. set E_1 of ∞-weighted edges along a single ray:
   $E_1 = \{(v_{i,j,k}, v_{i,j,k-1}) \mid i \in [1..n],\ j \in [1..l],\ k \in [2..m]\}$
2. set $E_2 = E_{2A} \cup E_{2B} \cup E_{2C} \cup E_{2D}$ of ∞-weighted edges between neighbored rays within a plane:
   $E_{2A} = \{(v_{i,j,k}, v_{i,j+1,max(0,k-\Delta_x)}) \mid i \in [1..n],\ j \in [1..l-1],\ k \in [1..m]\}$
   $E_{2B} = \{(v_{i,j,k}, v_{i,j-1,max(0,k-\Delta_x)}) \mid i \in [1..n],\ j \in [2..l],\ k \in [1..m]\}$

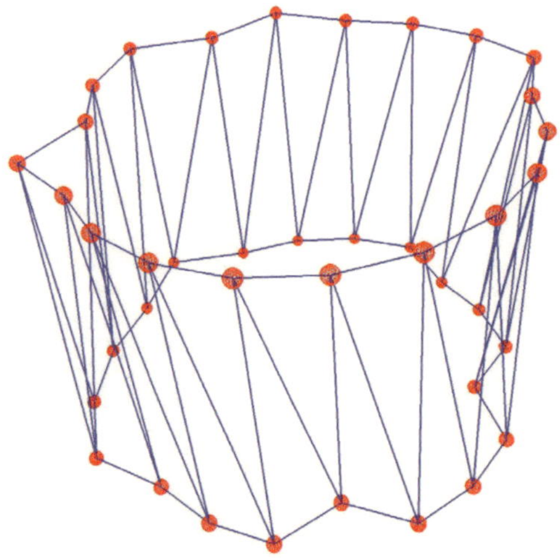

Fig. 9. Triangulation scheme for two neighbored evaluation planes.

$E_{2C} = \{(v_{i,1,k}, v_{i,l,max(0,k-\Delta_x)}) \mid i \in [1..n],\ k \in [1..m]\}$
$E_{2D} = \{(v_{i,l,k}, v_{i,0,max(0,k-\Delta_x)}) \mid i \in [1..n],\ k \in [1..m]\}$

3. set $E_3 = E_{3A} \cup E_{3B}$ of ∞-weighted edges between neighbored planes:
   $E_{3A} = \{(v_{i,j,k}, v_{i+1,j,max(0,k-\Delta_z)}) \mid i \in [1..n-1],\ j \in [1..l],\ k \in [1..m]\}$
   $E_{3B} = \{(v_{i,j,k}, v_{i-1,j,max(0,k-\Delta_z)}) \mid i \in [2..n],\ j \in [1..l],\ k \in [1..m]\}$
4. set $E_{st} = E_{source1} \cup E_{source2} \cup E_{sink1} \cup E_{sink2}$ of individually w-weighted edges to source and sink:
   $E_{source1} = \{(v_{i,j,1}, v_{source}) \mid i \in [1..n],\ j \in [1..l]\}$ with $w(i,j,1) = c(i,j,1)$
   $E_{sink1} = \{(v_{i,j,m}, v_{sink}) \mid i \in [1..n],\ j \in [1..l]\}$ with $w(i,j,m) = c(i,j,m)$
   $E_{source2} = \{(v_{i,j,k}, v_{source}) \mid i \in [1..n],\ j \in [1..l],\ k \in [2..m-1], c(v_{i,j,k}) - c(v_{i,j,k-1}) \geq 0\}$ with $w(i,j,k) = |c(v_{i,j,k}) - c(v_{i,j,k-1})|$
   $E_{sink2} = \{(v_{i,j,k}, v_{sink}) \mid i \in [1..n],\ j \in [1..l],\ k \in [2..m-1], c(v_{i,j,k}) - c(v_{i,j,k-1}) < 0\}$ with $w(i,j,k) = |c(v_{i,j,k}) - c(v_{i,j,k-1})|$

The edges along the single rays ensure that all nodes below the surface are included to form a closed set. Thereby the interior of the fiber bundle can be separated form the exterior. The edges connecting different rays and planes constrain the set of possible segmentations. The two parameters Δ_x and Δ_z used for edge construction (see E_2 and E_3) enforce smoothness and stiffness of the result. The greater the parameters get, the greater is the number of possible segmentations.

After the graph construction, the minimal cost closed set is computed on the graph via a polynomial time s-t-cut (Boykov & Kolmogorov, 2001), creating an optimal segmentation of the fiber bundle, delivering a point set containing a boundary point for each ray of each plane. For comparison and evaluation a closed surface/volume of the segmented fiber bundle is needed. Due to the ordering of the point set given by the ordered construction of planes and rays, the point cloud can be triangulated easily. Therefore, neighbored contour point sets are triangulated like shown in Fig. 9. For volume construction the triangulated surface can be voxelized.

Fig. 10. Samples of an ODF visualization. The colors encode the directions, green: anterior/posterior, blue: cranial/caudal, red: lateral.

With the help of this surface/volume construction a comparison with other segmentation algorithms is possible. Also the evaluation of segmentation quality becomes possible by the use of phantoms with defined fiber tracts and corresponding masks for comparison like done in (Bauer et al., 2010) for example with the help of the Dice Similarity Coefficient (Zou et al., 2004).

6. Visualizing the Fiber Orientation Distribution Function

DTI does not provide a good basis for resolving fiber crossings or fiber kissings within a certain voxel due to underlying tensor model. Advanced approaches like q-space imaging may overcome this problem, however, the corresponding acquisition technique needs large field gradients and time-consuming sampling steps. Thus, these approaches are rarely used for clinical tasks. Q-Ball imaging (Tuch, 2004) tries to overcome this problem and reconstructs the HARDI signal model independently. Instead of minimizing a function of variables arising from a model, the orientation distribution function (ODF) is calculated directly from the signal by a Fourier transformation and a projection, which is actually approximated by the Funk-Radon-transform. The correct calculation assumes a gradient which approximates a δ -distribution in time. Another possibility to reconstruct the ODF model-independently is to use spherical deconvolution (Tournier et al., 2004).
Fig. 10 shows ODF visualizations which may support the clinicians by assessing the uncertainty in the data and the fiber tracking algorithm. Because of not knowing the value of the ODF between the evaluated directions it is rather difficult to visualize the ODF as a surface without calculating many reconstruction points.
Our basic idea for visualizing an ODF is to map the reconstruction points to spherical coordinates by $(\varphi, \theta) \in [0, 2\pi] \times [0, \pi]$, which are afterwards inserted into a quadtree. The geometry of the quadtree can be used to build up a triangulation where the triangulation is refined at points with a high curvature of the corresponding surface. For that purpose, we split the quad tree according to the geodesic distances of two inserted reconstruction points on the sphere. Then, the algorithm can be formulated as follows:

1. Transform all reconstruction points in spherical coordinates via $\phi : S^2 \to \mathbf{R}^3, (x, y, z) \mapsto \left(\cos^{-1}(z/r), \text{atan2}(y, x), 0\right)$, where $r := \sqrt{x^2 + y^2 + z^2}$ and $S^2 := \left\{(x, y, z) \in \mathbf{R}^3 : \sqrt{x^2 + y^2 + z^2} = 1\right\}$

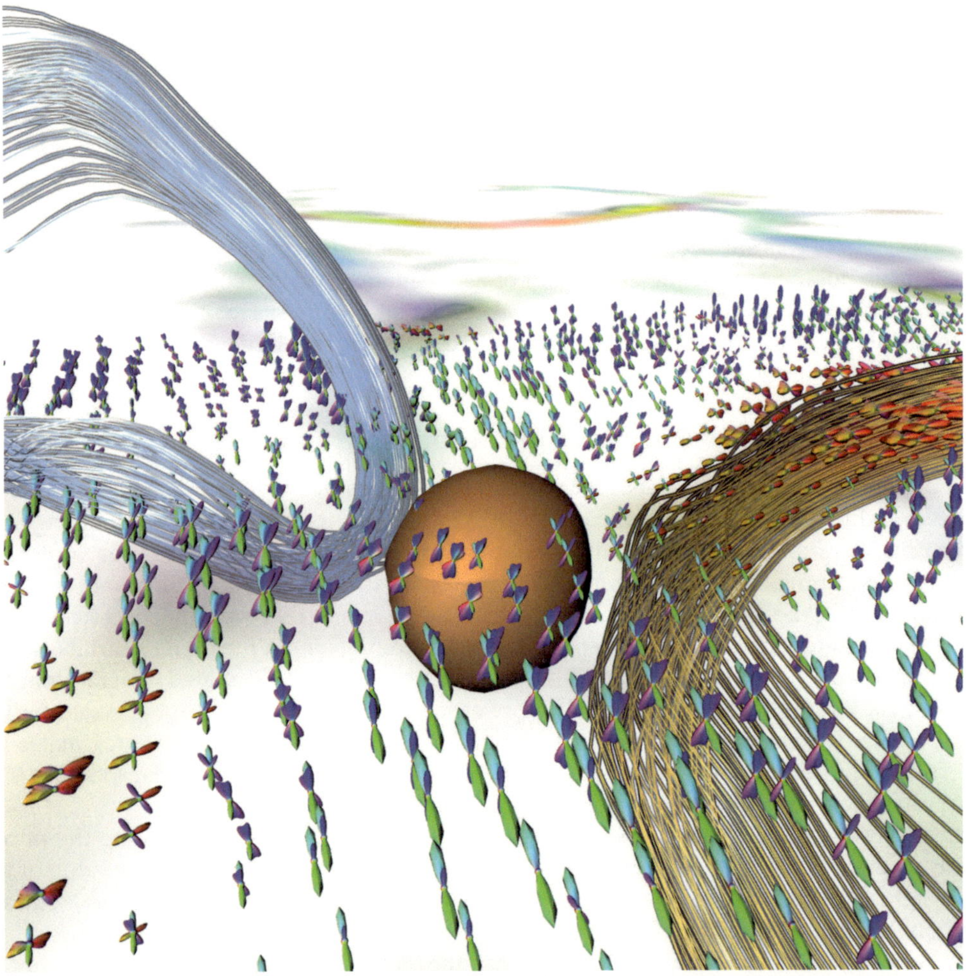

Fig. 11. Axial slice through the corpus callosum. The uncertainty of the fiber reconstruction can be assessed by visualizing the fiber orientation distribution function (fODF), which is a probability distribution on a sphere. The colors encode the directions, green: anterior/posterior, blue: cranial/caudal, red: lateral.

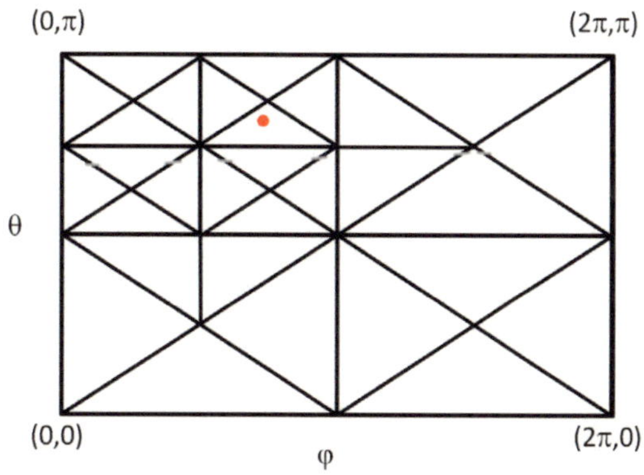

Fig. 12. Quad tree containing the adaptive triangulation of the plane. The cross marks an inserted direction. φ is on the x-axis and θ on the y-axis.

2. Insert the reconstruction points d_i which have a diffusion which is more than σ away from the mean. Insertion means setting the z-component to the odf's value
3. Split the quad tree recursively until the bounding volumes have satisfied an error condition (this is in general a function $\epsilon\left(d_1, \delta_i, ...d_n, \delta_n\right) \mapsto \mathbf{R}^+$, where δ_i is the distance of the quad to the inserted direction d_i. For computing the distance, we use the minima of geodesic distances of the vertices and the mid point to the inserted reconstruction point.
4. Insert additional vertices to avoid visual artifacts. This is done if a neighbor bounding volume has been split more often.
5. Map the plane to a sphere via $\phi^{-1}\left(\theta, \varphi, r\right) \mapsto r\left(\cos\varphi \sin\theta, \sin\varphi \sin\theta, cos\theta\right)$

Using this algorithm, which considers the metric of a sphere, the splitting leads to a good triangulation, also for small radii (small diffusion).

7. Conclusion

Technical challenges like improved spatial resolution, whole brain coverage, signal to noise ratio, or magnetic susceptibility artifacts constitute the basis for reliable quantification techniques in diffusion neuroimaging. For example, high-resolution 3D imaging sequences facilitated by parallel imaging will strongly contribute towards quantitative reliability. Still, in most cases, partial volume modeling will be key to yield highly reliable quantitative measurements due to the complexity or small spatial extent of both anatomical features and pathological alterations. For example, there is increasing evidence that subtle or even significant gray matter alterations play an important role in MS pathology (Zivadinov & Cox, 2007). Furthermore, preprocessing algorithms for registration, regularization, or outlier rejection are substantial influencing factors.

In the case of quantitative DTI, the assumption of a Gaussian diffusion process may not be adequate in areas of complex fiber structures like crossing or kissing fibers not only for fiber reconstruction but also for quantitative assessment. This problem has recently been addressed by multiple-compartment models, diffusion spectrum imaging, spherical deconvolution and persistent angular structure MRI (PAS-MRI), where higher order tensors or probability distributions describe the actual diffusion process. (Assaf et al., 2002) have already shown that

with q-space imaging the difference of values in the normal appearing white matter of patients with multiple sclerosis is more pronounced than with DTI. However, virtually all techniques based on HARDI data are still in an early state and are subject to improvement with respect to acquisition and postprocessing time so that they become useful for clinical routine.
We have given several examples in the context of diffusion neuroimaging where quantification techniques play an important role and have presented and discussed software and hardware phantoms for measuring their precision and reliability. Without such evaluation basis, several pitfalls and systematic errors might remain undetected.

8. References

Assaf, Y. & Basser, P. J. (2005). Composite hindered and restricted model of diffusion (CHARMED) MR imaging of the human brain, *Neuroimage* **27**: 48–58.

Assaf, Y., Ben-Bashat, D., Chapman, J., Peled, S., Biton, I., Kafri, M., Segev, Y., Hendler, T., Korczyn, A., Graif, M. & Cohen, Y. (2002). High b-value q-space analyzed diffusion-weighted mri: Application to multiple sclerosis, *Magnetic Resonance in Medicine* **47**(1): 115–126.

Assaf, Y., Freidlin, R. Z., Rohde, G. K. & Basser, P. J. (2004). New modeling and experimental framework to characterize hindered and restricted water diffusion in brain white matter, *Magn. Reson. Med.* **52**: 965–978.

Barboriak, D. (2003). Imaging of brain tumors with diffusion-weighted and diffusion tensor mr imaging, *Magn Reson Imaging Clin N Am* **11**: 379–401.

Basser, P. & Pajevic, S. (2003). Dealing with uncertainty in diffusion tensor MR data, *Israel Journal of Chemistry* **43**: 129–144.

Basser, P., Pajevic, S., Pierpaoli, C. & Aldroubi, A. (2002). Fiber tract following in the human brain using dt-mri data, *IEICE Trans. Inf. & Syst.* **E85-D**(1): 15–21.

Bauer, M. H. A., Egger, J., Barbieri, S., Klein, J., Freisleben, B., Hahn, H.-K. & Nimsky, C. (2010). A Fast and Robust Graph-based Approach for Boundary Estimation of Fiber Bundles Relying on Fractional Anisotropy Maps, *Proceedings of the 20th International Conference on Pattern Recognition (ICPR)*, Istanbul, Turkey, p. (to appear).

Behrens, T., Woolrich, M., Jenkinson, M., Johansen-Berg, H., Nunes, R., Clare, S., Matthews, P., Brady, J. & Smith, S. (2003). Characterization and propagation of uncertainty in diffusion-weighted mr imaging, *Magnetic Resonance in Medicine* **50**: 1077–1088.

Berman, J. I., Nagarajan, S. S., Berger, M. S. & Henry, R. G. (2004). Comparison of fiber tracking techniques in combination with functional localization in brain tumor patients, *Proceeding of ISMRM*, p. 1260.

Bhagat, Y. A. & Beaulieu, C. (2004). Diffusion anisotropy in subcortical white matter and cortical gray matter: Changes with aging and the role of CSF-suppression, *Magn. Reson. Imaging* **20**: 216–227.

Boykov, Y. & Kolmogorov, V. (2001). An Experimental Comparison of Min-Cut/Max-Flow Algorithms for Energy Minimization in Vision, *IEEE Transactions on Pattern Analysis and Machine Intelligence* **26**: 359–374.

Bra (n.d.). Project URL: `http://www.bic.mni.mcgill.ca/brainweb/`.

Chung, S., Lu, Y. & Henry, R. G. (2006). Comparison of bootstrap approaches for estimation of uncertainties of dti parameters, *NeuroImage* **33**(2): 531 – 541.

Collins, A., Zijdenbos, A., Kollokian, V., Sled, J., Kabani, N., Holmes, C. & Evans, A. (1998). Design and construction of a realistic digital brain phantom, *IEEE Trans. Med. Imaging* **17**(3): 463–468.

Egger, J., Freisleben, B., Setser, R., Renapuraar, R., Biermann, C. & O'Donnell, T. (2009). Aorta Segmentation for Stent Simulation, *12th International Conference on MICCAI, Cardiovascular Interventional Imaging and Biophysical Modelling Workshop*, London, United Kingdom.

Egger, J., O'Donnell, T., Hopfgartner, C. & Freisleben, B. (2008). Graph-Based Tracking Method for Aortic Thrombus Segmentation, *Proceedings of 4th European Congress for Medical and Biomedical Engineering, Engineering for Health*, Antwerp, Belgium.

Fieremans, E., De Deene, Y., Delputte, S., Ozdemir, M., Achten, E. & Lemahieu, I. (2008). The design of anisotropic diffusion phantoms for the validation of diffusion weighted magnetic resonance imaging, *Physics in Medicine and Biology* **53**: 5405–5419.

Fieremans, E., De Deene, Y., Delputte, S., Ozdemir, M., D'Asseler, Y., Vlassenbroeck, J., Deblaere, K., Achten, E. & Lemahieu, I. (2008). Simulation and experimental verification of the diffusion in an anisotropic fiber phantom, *J. Magn. Reson.* **190**(1): 189–199.

Fink, F., Klein, J., Lanz, M., Mitrovics, T., Lentschig, M., Hahn, H. K. & Hildebrandt, H. (2009). Comparison of diffusion tensor-based tractography and quantified brain atrophy for analyzing demyelination and axonal loss in ms., *J Neuroimaging* .

Friman, O., Farnebäck, G. & Westin, C.-F. (2006). A Bayesian approach for stochastic white matter tractography, *IEEE Transactions on Medical Imaging* **25**(8): 965–978.

Gössl, C., Fahrmeir, L., Pütz, B., Auer, L. & Auer, D. (2002). Fiber tracking from DTI using linear state space models: Detectability of the pyramidal tract, *Neuroimage* **16**: 378–388.

Griffin, C., Chard, D., Ciccarelli, O., Kapoor, R., Barker, G., Thompson, A. & Miller, D. (2001). Diffusion tensor imaging in early relapsing-remitting multiple sclerosis, *Multiple Sclerosis* **7**(5): 290–297.

Gössl, C., Fahrmeir, L., Pütz, B., Auer, L. & Auer, D. (2002). Fiber tracking from dti using linear state space models: detectability of the pyramidal tract, *Neuroimage* **16**(2): 378–388.

Gudbjartsson, H. & Patz, S. (1995). The Rician distribution of noisy MRI data, *Magn. Reson. Med.* **34**: 910–914.

Hahn, H. K., Klein, J., Nimsky, C., Rexilius, J. & Peitgen, H.-O. (2006). Uncertainty in diffusion tensor based fibre tracking, *Acta Neurochir Suppl* **98**: 33–41.

Heiervang, E., Behrens, T., Mackay, C., Robson, M. & Johansen-Berg, H. (2006). Between session reproducibility and between subject variability of diffusion mr and tractography measures, *Neuroimage* **33**(3): 867–77. 1053-8119 (Print)Journal Article.

Holmes, C., Hoge, R., Collins, D., Woods, R., Toga, A. & Evans, A. (1998). Enhancement of MR images using registration for signal averaging, *J. Comput. Assist. Tomogr.* **22**: 324–333.

Inglis, B., Neubauer, D., Yang, L., Plant, D., Mareci, T. & Muir, D. (1999). Diffusion tensor mr imaging and comparative histology of glioma engrafted in the rat spinal cord, *AJNR Am J Neuroradiol* **20**: 713–716.

Jones, D. (2003). Determining and visualizing uncertainty in estimates of fiber orientation from diffusion tensor MRI, *Magnetic Resonance in Medicine* **49**: 7–12.

Jones, D., Travis, A., Eden, G., Pierpaoli, C. & Basser, P. (2005). PASTA: Pointwise assessment of streamline tractography attributes, *Magn. Reson. Med.* **53**: 1462–1467.

Klein, J., Grötsch, A., Betz, D., Barbieri, S., Friman, O., Stieltjes, B., Hildebrandt, H. & Hahn, H. K. (2010). Qualitative and quantitative analysis of probabilistic and deterministic fiber tracking, *Medical Imaging 2010: Image Processing*, Vol. 7623, SPIE, pp. 76232A–1 – 76232A–8.

Klein, J., Hermann, S., Konrad, O., Hahn, H. K. & Peitgen, H.-O. (2007). Automatic Quantification of DTI Parameters along Fiber Bundles, *Proceeding of Image Processing for Medicine (BVM 2007)*, pp. 272–2.

Leemans, A., Sijbers, J., Verhoye, M., van der Linden, A. & van Dyck, D. (2005). Mathematical framework for simulating diffusion tensor mr neural fiber bundles, *Magnetic resonance in medicine* **53**(4): 944–953.

Li, K., Wu, X., Chen, D. Z. & Sonka, M. (2004a). Efficient optimal surface detection: theory, implementation, and experimental validation, *Society of Photo-Optical Instrumentation Engineers (SPIE) Conference Series*, Vol. 5370 of *Presented at the Society of Photo-Optical Instrumentation Engineers (SPIE) Conference*, pp. 620–627.

Li, K., Wu, X., Chen, D. Z. & Sonka, M. (2004b). Globally Optimal Segmentation of Interacting Surfaces with Geometric Constraints, *Proceedings of the IEEE CS Conf. Computer Vision and Pattern Recognition (CVPR)*, Vol. 1, pp. 394–399.

Li, K., Wu, X., Chen, D. Z. & Sonka, M. (2006). Optimal Surface Segmentation in Volumetric Images-A Graph-Theoretic Approach, *IEEE Transactions on Pattern Analysis and Machine Intelligence* **28**(1): 119–134.

Lin, C.-P., Tseng, W.-Y. I., Cheng, H.-C. & Chen, J.-H. (2001). Validation of diffusion tensor magnetic resonance axonal fiber imaging with registered manganese-enhanced optic tracts, *Neuroimage* **14**: 1035–1047.

Lori, N., Akbudak, E., Shimony, J., Cull, T., Snyder, A., Guillory, R. & Conturo, T. (2002). Diffusion tensor fiber tracking of human brain connectivity: acquisition methods, reliability analysis and biological results, *NMR Biomed.* **15**: 493–515.

McGraw, T. & Nadar, M. (2007). Stochastic dt-mri connectivity mapping on the gpu, *IEEE Trans. Vis. Comput. Graph.* **13**(6): 1504–1511.

Merhof, D., Hastreiter, P., Nimsky, C., Fahlbusch, R. & Greiner, G. (2005). Directional Volume Growing for the Extraction of White Matter Tracts from Diffusion Tensor Data, *SPIE - Medical Imaging 2005: Visualization, Image-Guided Procedures, and Display.*, Vol. 5744, pp. 165–172.

MeVisLab 2.0 (2010). Homepage at: http://www.mevislab.de.
URL: *http://www.mevislab.de*

Mori, S., Crain, B., Chacko, V. & van Zijl, P. (1999). Three-dimensional tracking of axonal projections in the brain by magnetic resonance imaging, *Ann Neurol.* **45**(2): 265–269.

Nimsky, C., Ganslandt, O., Hastreiter, P., Wang, R., Benner, T., Sorensen, A. G. & Fahlbusch, R. (2005). Preoperative and intraoperative diffusion tensor imaging-based fiber tracking in glioma surgery, *Neurosurgery* **56**(1): 130–138.

Oguz, I., Niethammer, M., Cates, J., Whitaker, R., Fletcher, T., Vachet, C. & Styner, M. (2009). Cortical correspondence with probabilistic fiber connectivity, *IPMI '09: Proceedings of the 21st International Conference on Information Processing in Medical Imaging*, Springer-Verlag, Berlin, Heidelberg, pp. 651–663.

Partridge, S., Mukherjee, P., Henry, R., Miller, S., Berman, J., Jin, H., Lu, Y., Glenn, O., Ferriero, D., Barkovich, A. & Vigneron, D. (2004). Diffusion tensor imaging: serial quantitation of white matter tract maturity in premature newborns, *Neuroimage* **22**: 1302–1314.

Pierpaoli, C., Jezzard, P., Basser, P., Barnett, A. & Di Chiro, G. (1996). Diffusion tensor MR imaging of the human brain, *Radiology* **201**: 637–648.

Pul, C., Buijs, J., Vilanova, A., Roos, F. & Wijn, P. (2006). Fiber tracking in newborns with perinatal hypoxic-ischemia at birth and at 3 months, *Radiology* **240**(1): 203–214.

Schlueter, M., Konrad, O., Hahn, H. K., Stieltjes, B., Rexilius, J. & Peitgen, H.-O. (2005). White matter lesion phantom for diffusion tensor data and its application to the assessment of fiber tracking, *Medical Imaging: Image Processing* **5746**: 835–844.

Tournier, J.-D., Calamante, F., Gadian, D. G. & Connelly, A. (2004). Direct estimation of the fiber orientation density function from diffusion-weighted mri data using spherical deconvolution, *NeuroImage* **23**(3): 1176 – 1185.

Tournier, J.-D., Yeh, C.-H., Calamante, F., Cho, K.-H., Connelly, A. & Lin, C.-P. (2008). Resolving crossing fibres using constrained spherical deconvolution: Validation using diffusion-weighted imaging phantom data, *Neuroimage* **42**(2): 617–625.

Tuch, D. (2004). Q-ball imaging, *Magnetic Resonance in Medicine* **52**: 1358–1372.

Weinstein, D. M., Kindlmann, G. L. & Lundberg, E. C. (1999). Tensorlines: Advection-diffusion based propagation through diffusion tensor fields, *VISUALIZATION '99: Proceedings of the 10th IEEE Visualization 1999 Conference (VIS '99)*, IEEE Computer Society, Washington, DC, USA, pp. 249–253.

Wu, X. & Chen, D. Z. (2002). Optimal Net Surface Problems with Applications, *Proceedings of the 29th International Colloquium on Automata, Languages and Programming (ICALP)*, Malaga, Spain, pp. 1029–1042.

Zivadinov, R. & Cox, J. (2007). Neuroimaging in multiple sclerosis, *Int Rev Neurobiol* **79**: 449–474.

Zou, K. H., Warfield, S. K., Bharatha, A., Tempany, C. M. C., Kaus, M. R., Haker, S. J., Wells, W. M., Jolesz, F. A. & Kikinis, R. (2004). Statistical Validation of Image Segmentation Quality Based on a Spatial Overlap Index, *Academic Radiology* **11**(2): 178–189.

2

Exploring brain circuitry: Simultaneous application of Transcranial Magnetic Stimulation and functional Magnetic Resonance Imaging

Elisabeth de Castro Caparelli, Ph.D.
Brookhaven National Laboratory, NY and Stony Brook University, NY USA

1. Introduction

Transcranial magnetic stimulation (TMS) has proven invaluable as a technique for stimulating specific brain areas; such local stimulation induces changes in cortical excitability, and modifies specific cognitive functions. Hence, it affords a good measure of a variety of parameters, including neural conduction and processing time, activation thresholds, and facilitation and inhibition in the brain's cortex, so supporting the exploration of human motor- and visual-systems, and cognition. This technique has been widely used as a research tool to investigate the brain's plasticity, response to emotions, and cognition. It also has been used as a clinical tool to study some neurological diseases, such as epilepsy, and often as a treatment tool in alleviating psychiatric disorders, and for hastening recovery of motor function after stroke.

Functional magnetic resonance imaging (fMRI), based on Blood Oxygenation Level Dependence (BOLD) contrast, is one of the commonest neuroimaging techniques. The preference for this imaging modality rests upon its ability to "record", non-invasively, neuronal activity when the human brain is involved in specific tasks. Furthermore, because it carries low risk or none, and lacks side effects, experiments can be repeated and verified. Due to these advantages, BOLD-fMRI has been used in studies that involve healthy populations, people with diseases, and those using drugs, to explore the brain activity during primary and higher cognitive/behavioral tasks, using a variety of different paradigms, to evaluate attention, memory, language processing, and decision-making.

These two techniques have been widely used in neuroscience, mainly because of their non-invasiveness and low risk factor; however, using them alone has revealed some limitations. For example, because the stimulation paradigms used in fMRI studies are complex, it is unclear whether or not a specific area is essential for a particular function; moreover, the resulting map of brain functional connectivity, based on cross-correlating the BOLD signal, is an indirect measurement and, hence, the direction of causality remains uncertain. Similarly, TMS rests on the implicit assumption that the applied magnetic pulse locally disrupts neural activity at the site of stimulation, inducing changes in the corresponding behavioral performance. However, recent TMS-fMRI studies indicated that the neural consequences of focal TMS are not restricted to the site of stimulation, but spread throughout different brain regions. Therefore, the only reliable way directly to assess the neural effects of a TMS stimulus is via the simultaneous combination of TMS and functional brain-imaging techniques. Particularly, the coincident TMS-fMRI combination allows us to stimulate brain circuits while simultaneously monitoring changes in its activity and behavior. Such an approach can help to identify brain networks of functional relevance, and support causal brain-behavior inferences across the entire brain. Undoubtedly, this approach promises to contribute majorly to cognitive neuroscience. However, the drawback to its universal adoption is the great technical challenge that this technique imposes, and, thus, few research groups routinely employ it.

In this chapter, I overview the principles underlying the fMRI and TMS techniques, discuss the general applications of each, and detail the safety issues related to using TMS. Thereafter, I describe the technical implementation of the TMS device inside the MRI scanners, and finally outline the current possibilities and limitations of this promising multimodality technique.

2. fMRI Overview

Basis

fMRI is a non-ionizing, non-invasive imaging technique that allows us to use information generated by the hemodynamic process to study brain function. Although the connection between neural activity and changes in blood flow and blood oxygenation in the human brain was known since the end of nineteen century (Roy, et al. 1890), it was only toward the end of the twentieth century that this phenomena started to be explored.

The hemodynamic response is defined as the dynamic regulation of the blood flow in the brain. Thus, when neurons perform some specific task, their consumption of oxygen increases and because they do not accumulate internal energy reserves, viz. glucose and oxygen, they require the rapid delivery of energy as they start firing. Consequently, after a delay of about 1–5 seconds, local blood flow increases and rises to a peak over 4–5 seconds before falling back to baseline (Raichle, et al. 2006); since this increase in blood supply exceeds the local increase in oxygen consumption, there is a local change in blood flow and oxygenation (Fox, et al. 1985).

Such changes induce temporary modifications in tissue permeability, so altering the MRI signal. Essentially, since hemoglobin is diamagnetic when oxygenated (oxyhemoglobin) but paramagnetic when deoxygenated (deoxihemoglobin) (Pauling, et al. 1936) the magnetic resonance (MR) signal of blood differs slightly, depending on the oxygenation level. More specifically, the effective transverse relaxation time (T_2*) increases in activated brain regions with decreased deoxyhemoglobin concentration (Ogawa, et al. 1990) that causes a local increase of the MRI signal (Fig. 1). This effect, called the blood oxygenation level dependence (BOLD) contrast, is the basis for most fMRI studies.

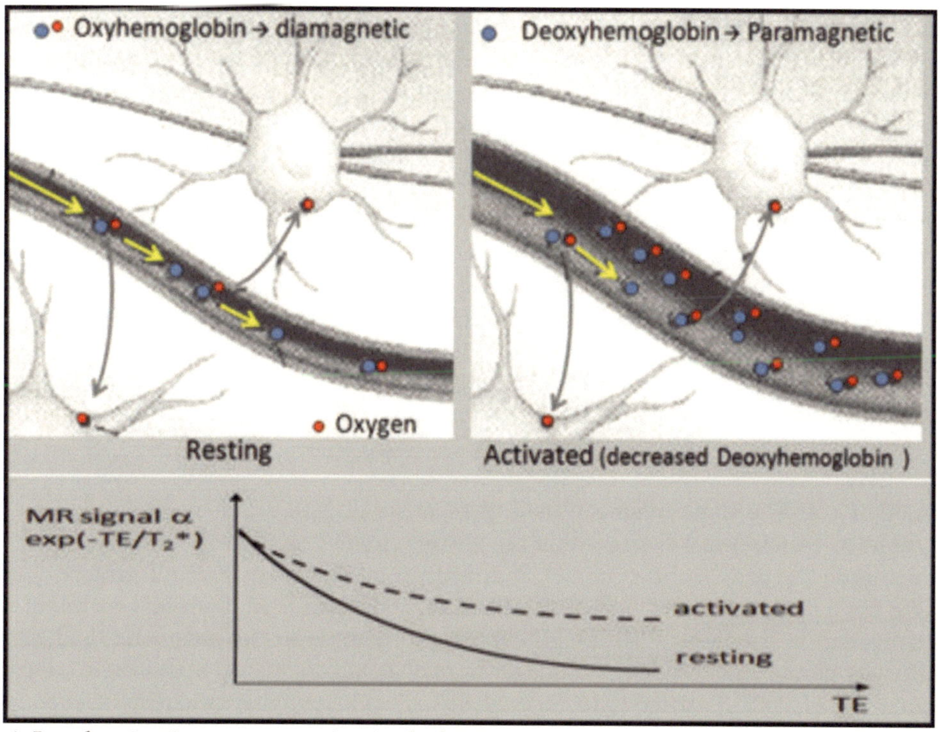

Fig. 1. Local activation versus resting in the brain.

Changes in BOLD contrast can be observed by collecting data in an MRI scanner with sequence parameters sensitive to changes in magnetic susceptibility, i.e., by using T_2* sensitive imaging and fast sequences, such as Echo Planar Imaging (EPI) (Bandettini, et al. 1992). These changes can be either positive or negative depending on the relative changes in both cerebral blood flow (CBF) and oxygen consumption. Increases in CBF that exceed changes in oxygen consumption will entail an increased BOLD signal (activation); conversely, decreases in CBF that surpass changes in oxygen consumption will engender a decreased one (deactivation). Since the BOLD contrast-to-noise ratio (CNR) increases with the static magnetic field (Gati, et al. 1997, Okada, et al. 2005) recent technical improvements, such as using high magnetic fields (van der Zwaag, et al. 2009) and multichannel RF reception (Pruessmann, et al. 1999), have advanced spatial resolution to the millimeter scale. Currently functional images are usually acquired every 1-4 seconds with a spatial resolution of 2-4 millimeters on each side of the cubic voxel.

Despite hardware and software improvements to increase the signal-to-noise ratio (SNR) the BOLD signal is still very small (typically 1-5%) (Caparelli, et al. 2003). Furthermore, because of the significant intra/inter subject variability, we cannot directly quantify fMRI results. Accordingly, the data must be evaluated statistically, which involves many experimental repetitions of a thought, action, or experience to determine reliably which areas of the brain are activated/deactivated.

Data analysis: The goal of fMRI data analysis is to reveal correlations between brain activation and the task performed by a person during the scan. However, the BOLD signal is small, and other sources of noise in the acquired data, such as small head motion, and physiological noise, can mask the results; hence , the data must be corrected to eliminate these unwanted effects. Accordingly, after reconstructing the resulting series of 3D images of the brain, the output of the scanning session undergoes a series of steps starting with correction for motion. Following this, the data is normalized to put all the images in the same frame for a group analysis. This step puts all images for each subject into one standard format that is set by a template; finally spatial filtering is also performed. The final outcome is a time series of 3 D scanned volumes ready to be correlated with the used task voxel-by-voxel, which will produce a statistical map of task-dependent activation.

There are many software packages available for the statistical analysis of the fMRI data, such as, the Statistical Parametric Mapping (SPM) (Friston 1996), Analysis of Functional NeuroImages (AFNI) (Cox 1996), FMRIB Software Library (FSL) (Smith, et al. 2004), and most of them also offers the data pre-processing described above.

MRI Safety

Magnetic field: The static magnetic field, present in all MRI scanners (example fig. 2), is generated by the electrical currents that are always circulating the superconductor material that compose the MRI scanner tunnel; it is used to align the spin of all protons (^1H) by making them move around an axis along the direction of the field, thereby generating a net magnetization in the tissue. Although exposure of people to this magnetic field has not resulted in permanent biological damage, it may entail in them a transient dizziness (Chakeres, et al. 2005), vertigo (Glover, et al. 2007), and a metallic taste (Cavin, et al. 2007). This field can also interfere with the function of electromechanical devices, and attract any iron-containing (ferromagnetic) objects, making them move suddenly and with great force into the scanner, thereby posing in risk anyone who is in the projectile's (metallic "flying" object) path. The magnetic field can also exert a pull on any ferromagnetic object in the body, such as certain medication pumps or aneurysm clips, causing serious internal body damages.

Therefore, any object that is brought to the scanner room needs to be MRI-compatible while everyone who will be inside or at the vicinity of an MRI scanner, viz., staff , patients, and study volunteers, must undergo a careful screening to avoid any incident that could lead to serious injuries and sometimes, even to death.

Radio frequency (RF): RF pulses alter the alignment of the net magnetization, causing the hydrogen nuclei to produce a rotating electromagnetic field that the receiver coil at the MRI scanner can detect. This RF pulse can heat living tissue to the point of inducing hyperthermia in patients/research volunteers; therefore, to avoid this problem, the specific absorption rate (SAR) parameter was established that determines how much RF a specific body can tolerate safely according to tissue density. SAR is defined as the power absorbed per mass of tissue, usually averaged over a specific volume, so providing a measure of the rate of absorbed energy by the tissue, in watts per kilogram, when exposed to a RF electromagnetic field (Oh, et al. 2010).

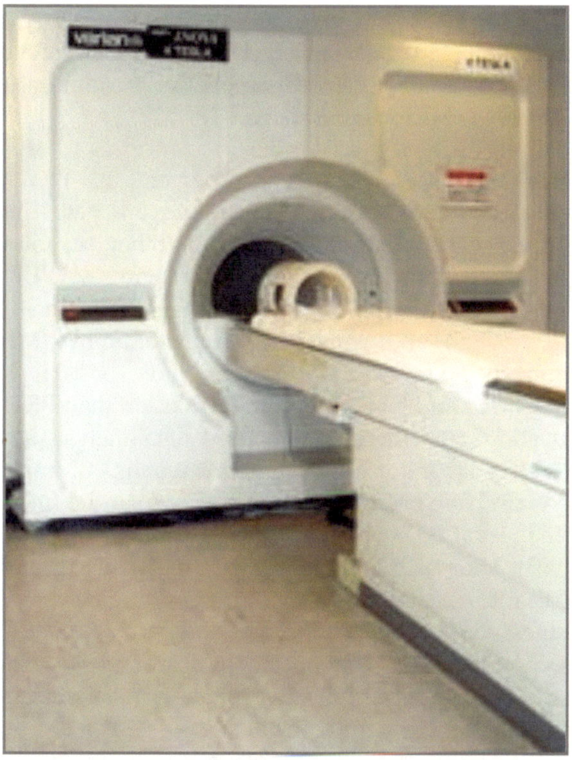

Fig. 2. 4 Tesla MRI Varian scanner at Brookhaven National Laboratory (BNL)

RF can also heat some tattoo pigments, particularly those that contain trace metals and are frequently used for regular tattoos or tattooed eye-liner (permanent makeup), potentially causing skin burns (Stecco, et al. 2007, Wagle, et al. 2000)

Peripheral nerve stimulation (PNS): Magnetic field gradients encode the spatial position of the MR signal generating an MR image. Special coils designed to produce a linearly varying spatial dependence of the magnetic field along a particular axis create these gradients. Fast sequences, mainly those commonly employed for some imaging techniques, such as fMRI, and Diffusion Tensor Imaging (DTI), require these fields to be switched on and off quickly. However, such rapid switching can causing peripheral nerve stimulation, inducing symptoms from mild tingling and muscle twitching to a sensation of pain. Indeed, volunteers have reported a twitching sensation, particularly in their extremities, when exposed to rapidly switched fields. Therefore to avoid PNS incidents, regulatory $d\mathbf{B}/dt$ (change in field per unit time) limits were specified (Glover 2009).

Acoustic noise: The exchanges between the readout and phase encoding currents in the gradient coils under the main static magnetic field of the MR scanner induce Lorentz forces that act on the gradient coils. Accordingly, the coils and wires buckle and bend, inducing compression waves in the surrounding gradient supports; these motions are conducted toward the MR system's peripheral structures and launched into air as loud acoustic noises (clicking or beeping). Because the Lorentz forces increase logarithmically with the magnetic fields' strength and with the applied gradient current, the noise levels rise with both. During echo planar imaging (EPI) the equivalent-continuous sound pressure levels (SPLs) range from 90–117 dB, with a peak level up to 130 dB at 1.5 T; at 3.0T, they range from 105–133 dB with a peak level up to 140 db (Moelker, et al. 2003). Therefore, using appropriate ear protection, such as MRI-compatible sound-suppressor headphones and ear plugs, is essential for anyone inside the MRI scanner room.

fMRI: Pluses & Pitfalls

fMRI is a neuroimage technique that offers several advantages: it noninvasively records brain signals without risks of radiation inherent in other scanning methods, such as computed tomography (CT) or positron emission tomography (PET) scans; it has high spatial resolution (2–3 mm) and records signals from all regions of the brain, unlike electroencephalography (EEG) and magnetoencephalography (MEG) that are biased towards the cortical surface; and, BOLD-fMRI offers better spatial resolution than EEG and MEG, and has similar spatial- and better temporal-resolution than PET. fMRI is widely used to image brain "activation" and there are standard data-analysis approaches that allow researchers from different laboratories to compare results. Cross-correlations of BOLD signal changes in the brain have been used to indirectly map the functional connectivity in the brain, including the visual (Ogawa, et al. 1992), motor (Kim, et al. 1993), and language areas (Hinke, et al. 1993). Thus, BOLD-fMRI is used extensively to study brain connectivity in humans due to MRI's intrinsically low risks.

However, the indirectness of the fMRI connectivity measurements is a concern because the postulated interconnection pathways rely on biophysical models (Friston, et al. 2003). The lack of specificity on the direct association between the standard stimulus paradigm and the corresponding activated areas (1 cognitive function => 1 specific brain area) is another limitation in traditional fMRI studies. Pernet and colleagues recently reviewed this issue (Pernet, et al. 2007), underlining the need to use several cognitive processes to categorize objects (e.g., related to information encoding, attention, and memory); thus, a generic effect of categorization could easily pass as a brain correlate of category specificity. The solution for this non-specificity problem entails a difficult theoretical consideration, attaining the appropriate dimensionality of the design is practically unfeasible, since a true demonstration of category specificity would require exhaustively testing all possible interactions between categories and task properties. Therefore, brain activation patterns consistent with category specificity remain unidentified. In addition, a category-specificity effect is not localized to a given processing region; instead, it concerns the strength of functional connection from one area to another. Thus, as suggested by these authors, only by testing the effective connectivity, i.e., by measuring the influence that one neuronal system or cortical area exerts over another we can understand the processes at work in each module, and assert the process/information interaction. Finally, because of the complexity of the stimulation paradigms used in functional studies, frequently involving many brain regions and more than one basic function, it is unclear whether or not a specific area is essential for a particular function (Pernet, et al. 2007, Tomasi, et al. 2007). Therefore, since fMRI findings are always correlations, the direction of causality cannot be determined.

The precise relationship between neural signals and BOLD is actively researched. In general, changes in BOLD signal correlate well with changes in blood flow. In fact, the BOLD signal represents sophisticated convolution of changes in the cerebral metabolic rate of oxygen (CMRO2), the CBF, and cerebral blood volume (CBV) associated with focal neuronal activity (i.e., the energy consumption of the neuronal population); therefore, it indirectly measures neuronal activity composed of CBF contributions from larger arteries and veins, smaller arterioles and venules, and capillaries. Experimental results indicate that the BOLD signal can be weighted to the smaller vessels, and hence, closer to the active neurons, by using alternative MRI techniques (Song, et al. 2003) or larger magnetic fields, since the size of the BOLD signal increases with the increase of the magnetic field's strength.

fMRI has poor temporal resolution because the BOLD response peaks approximately 5 seconds after neuronal firing begins in an area, and it is difficult to distinguish BOLD responses to different events that occur within a short time. Therefore, to overcome these drawbacks, some multimodalities are under development, such as combining fMRI signals having relatively high spatial resolution with signals recorded with other techniques, such as EEG or MEG with higher temporal resolution but worse spatial resolution.

3. Introduction to TMS

History of Transcranial Magnetic Stimulation

Even though Franz Mesmer, in the eighteen century, has proposed the use of magnets to cure disease, it was not until the end of nineteenth century that scientists started to use magnetic energy to alter brain activity. The first publications on magnetic stimulation described Jacques D'Arsonval's experiments in 1898 stimulating the retina, and similar work by Silvanus P. Thompson in 1910 (Thompson 1910); at that time, the magnetic stimulators were powerful enough to activate the retinal cells, causing the subjects to perceive light flashes, but the fields generated were too weak to stimulate brain tissue.

In 1965, Bickford and Fremming (Bickford, et al. 1965) used a damped 500 Hz sinusoidal magnetic field to demonstrate muscular stimulation in animals and humans. Subsequently, Oberg (1973) magnetically excited nerve tissue. Polson and colleagues, in 1982, reported the first successful magnetic stimulation of superficial nerves (Polson, et al. 1982). Finally, three years later, the first Transcranial magnetic stimulation of the central nervous system and cortical regions was achieved (Barker, et al. 1985). Neurologists quickly adopted Barker's device, and now routinely employ single-stimulus TMS instruments to measure nerve-conduction time. The therapeutic potential of TMS was unrealized until the repetitive stimulator (rTMS), which generates up to 30 pulses per second, became available in the 1990s.

Basis

TMS is based on the Faraday's principle of electromagnetic induction, wherein a pulse of current flowing through a coil of wire generates a magnetic field. According to the Biot-Savart law (Jackson 1965, Reitz, et al. 1993) when a electric current flows through a ferromagnetic material it generates a magnetic field that is perpendicular to the current's direction (Fig. 3). If this magnetic field varies with time, this field will induce a current in any conductive material nearby; the rate of change determines the size of the induced current (Faraday's law). Finally, by Lenz's law, this induced current always flows in a direction that will oppose the change in magnetic field causing it (Jackson 1965). This principle of electromagnetic induction describes how a brief, high-current magnetic pulse produced in a TMS coil induces a current on the brain region lying underneath the coil, resulting on the depolarization of the neurons (Hallett 2000, Sack, et al. 2003). However, the current induced in the brain is not composed of free electrons but of the ions, which are responsible for tissue conductivity.

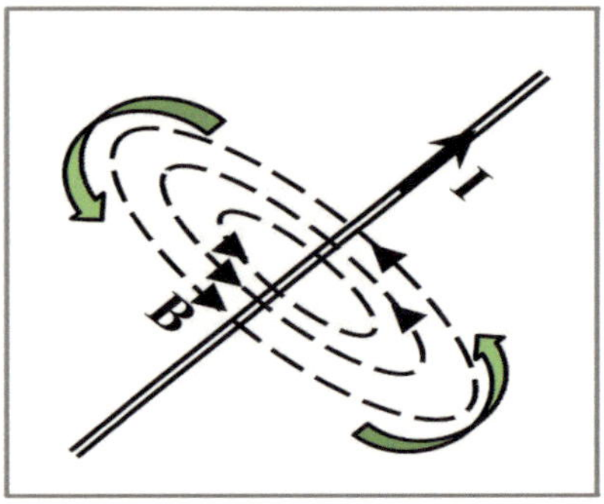

Fig. 3. Magnetic field lines, B, surrounding the current distribution, I,

TMS devices are made of two hardware components: a high-current pulse generator that produces discharge currents of about 5,000 amps (Figure 4 shows an example of the top-of-the- line instrument); and, a stimulating coil that generates magnetic pulses with field strengths of 1 -2 Tesla, and duration of 200 - 400 μs, depending on the coil shape/size. Fig 5a depicts the more traditional circular TMS coil shapes that produce pulses of high-intensity magnetic fields; however, they are not as focus as the figure-of-eight coil, shown in Fig. 5b, that can stimulate a region as small as 1 cm^2; however, this second coil shape is not as powerful as the circular coil (Anand, et al. 2002, Hallett 2000, Jalinouz 1998, Sack, et al. 2003). The pulses from coils shapes showed in Figure 5a and 5b can only penetrate the brain's cortical regions, about 1.5 cm beneath the scalp (Epstein, et al. 1990, Rudiak, et al. 1994, Wassermann 1998), but alternative shapes were developed, such as the double-cone coil, Fig. 5c, that was designed to stimulate brain structures down to 3 - 4 cm (Tada, et al. 1990).

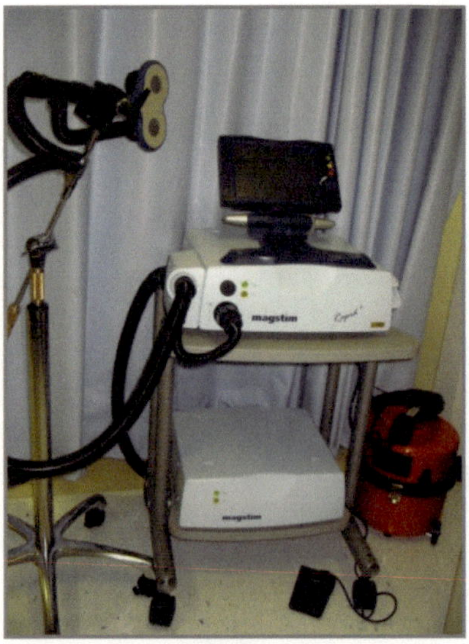

Fig. 4. Magstim super-rapid[2] TMS device at BNL that can deliver pulses reaching up to 100 Hz.

The TMS device can apply different stimulus intensities; for some cognitive functions, we can associate intensity with the ability to induce, or not, a specific behavioral output, which can define the threshold. For the motor area, the threshold for a motor-evoked potential (MEP) statistically is defined as the lowest intensity of stimulus needed to induce thumb movement, or to trigger MEPs of 50 mV or more in the abductor pollicis brevis muscle (thumb abductor muscle) for at least 50% of the applied pulses (Rostrup, et al. 1996, Sack, et al. 2003). Another observable output induced by TMS stimulus is the phosphene sensation. This feeling is characterized by experiencing flashes of light without light actually entering the eye; TMS induces this sensation in some people when the stimulus is applied on the occipital area. Thus, the phosphene threshold is defines as the lower intensity needed to generate the visualization of phosphenes when the stimulus is applied in the occipital area for at least 50% of the applied pulses (Stewart, et al. 2001).

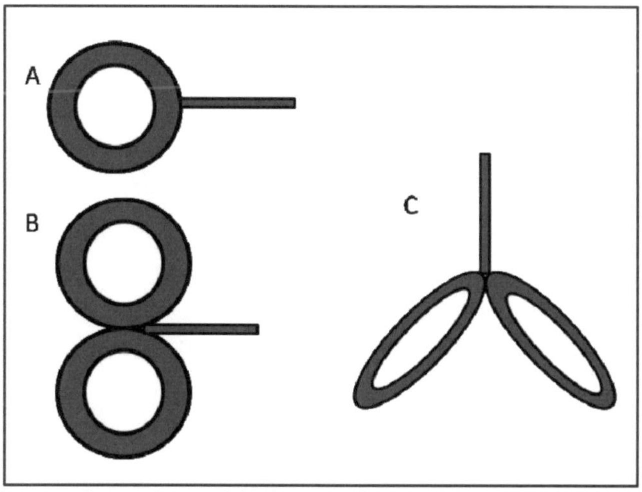

Fig. 5. TMS coil shapes: a) circular coil; b) figure-of-eight coil; c) double- cone coil

The TMS stimulus is also applied in several different protocols: as a single pulse, i.e., it is applied without repetition, generally to define or evaluate a stimulus threshold, or to disrupt a specific cognitive function; as a paired-pulse that is defined as a pair of TMS pulses applied consecutively from a single coil (one sub-threshold habituation pulse followed by a supra-threshold stimulus pulse) it is used to study intra-cortical inhibition and facilitation (Chen, et al. 1998, Kujirai, et al. 1993). For example, when TMS is delivered to motor cortex with an inter-stimulus interval of 1–4 ms, the first pulse suppresses the amplitude of the motor potential evoked by the second pulse, consistent with intracortical inhibition. However, with intervals of 8–15 ms, the second pulse evokes a larger motor potential than an equivalent single-pulse TMS, consistent with intra-cortical facilitation. Another common setup is the double-coil wherein the TMS pulse is applied simultaneously through two coils positioned in two different brain regions; it has been used for studying intra-cortical interactions and for comparing the processing times of different brain regions. Finally, the most powerful protocol for this technique is the repetitive TMS (rTMS) that generates a train of TMS pulses separated by intervals of less than 1 second, i.e., at frequencies that range from > 1 Hz up to 25 Hz in humans. Basically, the effects of rTMS pulses temporally summate, causing a greater change in neural activity than those changes induced by other protocols, and thereby offering a wide range of applications in basic neuroscience and as a clinical tool. For example, rTMS can induce changes in neurotransmitter systems and hormonal axes (Ben-Shachar, et al. 1997, Burt, et al. 2002, Keck, et al. 2000, Keck, et al. 2002, Kole, et al. 1999, Post, et al. 2001). It can also regulate the expression of some genes and the synthesis of some peptides that are important for neuronal plasticity and synaptic development (Keck, et al. 2000, Lisanby, et al. 2000, Schlaepfer, et al. 2004). Depending upon the intensity of the stimulus, rTMS either has anticonvulsant properties in epileptic patients, or reduces the threshold for seizure (Griskova, et al. 2006, Lisanby, et al. 2000, Wassermann, et al. 2001). rTMS is also used as a antidepressant treatment (Daskalakis, et al. 2008), and after significant positive results from numerous clinical trials, it was approved recently by the US Food and Drug Administration (FDA). Nevertheless, since rTMS can induce seizure, it poses some risk to people (Anand, et al. 2002).

Safety

Some safety issues are related to rTMS studies, mainly high-frequency protocols. Single-pulse TMS and low frequency rTMS (<1Hz) in healthy adults appears to carry little risk beyond occasionally causing local discomfort at the site of stimulation or a transient headache in susceptible subjects; no short- or long-term sequela have been described in safety studies with either modality in presumed normal adults (Anand, et al. 2002). Also, there have been no reports of ill effects after magnetic stimulation of the peripheral nervous system and, in the case of cortical stimulation, the incidence of side effects has been extremely low, and well within that expected numbers from statistics for various patient groups (Kandler 1990).

High frequency, high-intensity repetitive TMS (rTMS) carries some risk of inducing seizure even in normal subjects (Anand, et al. 2002, Wassermann 1998). In the ten years since research with TMS started (1985), there were seven documented accidental seizures. For this reason, a group of experts gathered in 1996 to review data on the safety of rTMS and to develop guidelines for its safe use; their findings were published in 1998(Wassermann 1998), detailing all possible rTMS risks and proposing safe guidelines to minimize them . Since then, rTMS risks declined considerably; ten years later a workshop held in Italy again reviewed the safety issues of TMS application; a summary was published in 2009 (Rossi, et al. 2009).

Unwanted long-term effects are also another important safety concern with TMS studies. Even though there are no registered long-term lasting effects for single-pulse TMS (Bridgers 1991, Chokroverty, et al. 1995),(Sack, et al. 2003) , some studies with high-frequency rTMS recorded mild effects persisting for about one hour after the TMS session (Flitman, et al. 1998, Little, et al. 2000, Triggs, et al. 1999), (Sack, et al. 2003). Hence, the first published guideline recommended some precautions with high frequency/intensities rTMS studies, for example, including a of pre- and post-neurological and/or neuropsychological examination, with another follow-up one (Wassermann 1998). Nevertheless there is no evidence of permanent, sustained negative sequelae of rTMS, and long-term cognitive- and neuropsychological-changes after single rTMS sessions are considered negligible in the second guideline based on the preceding bibliography. However, when cumulative daily

sessions of rTMS are administered therapeutically, the latest guideline strongly recommended employing neuropsychological monitoring (Rossi, et al. 2009).
Some TMS devices have received FDA approval for peripheral nerve stimulation; cortical stimulation remains investigational. Studies performed with TMS are classified in two groups: a) Non-significant risk (NSR), and, b) significant risk (SR). The former may only require an IRB-approved protocol and consent; SR studies additionally require FDA approval.

General applications

Since 1985, when the first TMS equipment was developed, TMS has been extensively used to explore aspects of human brain physiology in basic neuroscience, and in clinic applications. Initially TMS has shown to alter excitability thresholds and response latencies in several clinical circumstances, such as in people with certain diseases (Berardelli, et al. 1991) and those taking specific medications (Ziemann, et al. 1996). Thus, it was used to measure the cortical excitability thresholds in studies of epilepsy (Werhahn, et al. 2000)], and to improve motor conduction in patients with such deficits, viz., Parkinson's disease (Pascual-Leone, et al. 1994). Its application was also extended to studies of motor function in schizophrenic patients (Puri, et al. 1996), and for the prognosis of recovery from stroke (Rapisarda, et al. 1996). Treating depression was the major application of TMS (George, et al. 1995, George, et al. 1997, Pascual-Leone, et al. 1996); several years of clinical trials clearly demonstrated the value of this technique as an alternative treatment tool for patients who do not tolerate existing medications. Due to its great success, the FDA recently approved TMS for treating depression. TMS improves mood in depressive patients; accordingly, there was an increased interest in using TMS to clarify its effects on mood improvement that now is considered as a consequence of the production of neuroendocrine effect (Keck, et al. 2001). It was also verified recently that TMS can induce the stimulation of striatal dopamine release (Strafella, et al. 2001), the modulation of neurotransmiters (Keck, et al. 2000) and an increase of blood flow in the stimulated regions and connected areas (Speer, et al. 2000).
Researchers in the cognitive and behavioral neurosciences are exploring the ability of TMS to generate artificial lesions temporarily or to turn off the function of specific cortical regions, thereby allowing the functional identification of those brain areas more essential for a given task. Initials neuroscience studies with TMS were limited to animals or humans with pathological lesions; currently, researchers are extending their explorations to the healthy population. For instance, TMS is employed concurrently with some cognitive/behavioral tasks either to disrupt the execution of an specific task by perturbing some fundamental brain regions, or to improve performance by interrupting unimportant and/or competing brain signals (Walsh, et al. 1998). TMS impaired performance during learning and a spatial-memory task (Muri, et al. 1995), and suppressed visual perception during some visual tasks (Amassian, et al. 1989, Beckers, et al. 1995, Miller, et al. 1996), It also was used to investigate the effects of speech on the excitability of the corticospinal pathways of hand muscles (Tokimura, et al. 1996), and the response of transcallosal connections after magnetic stimulation compared with electrical stimulation(Cracco, et al. 1989). The system of callosal fibers activated by transcranial magnetic stimulation revealed the topography of fibers in the human corpus callosum mediating interhemispheric inhibition between the motor cortices (Meyer, et al. 1998). TMS was used to assess the plasticity of the cortical topography

in normal volunteers (Pascual-Leone, et al. 1994) and in patients suffering from stroke (Caramia, et al. 1996, Hamdy, et al. 1996) and amputations (Kew, et al. 1994).

4. The Simultaneous TMS & fMRI

The TMS technique rests on the implicit assumption that the induced magnetic stimulation locally disrupts neural activity at the site of stimulation, inducing changes in the correspondent behavioral performance. However, recent TMS-functional magnetic resonance imaging (fMRI) studies imply that the neural consequences of focal TMS are not restricted to the stimulation site (Bestmann, et al. 2003, Bestmann, et al. 2004, Ruff, et al. 2006, Ruff, et al. 2008), but spread throughout different brain regions. Accordingly, the only satisfactory way to directly assess the neural effects of a TMS stimulus is by simultaneously combining TMS and functional brain-imaging techniques(Sack 2006).
This combination opens up a new venue in neuroscience research. TMS supports a focused, controlled manipulation of neural activity, while the imaging techniques allow the functional evaluation of the brain's response to this local neuronal interference. Researchers have explored this multimodality combination of TMS and positron emission tomography (PET)(Paus, et al. 1997, Paus, et al. 1998), single-photon emission computed tomography (SPEC)(Fregni, et al. 2006)], electroencephalography (EEG) (Schutter, et al. 2006, Thut, et al. 2003), near- infrared spectroscopy (NIRS) (Hada, et al. 2006), fMRI (Bastings, et al. 1998, Boroojerdi, et al. 1999, Boroojerdi, et al. 2000, Devlin, et al. 2003, Roberts, et al. 1997), either simultaneously or in separated sections. However, because the simultaneous combination of TMS and fMRI is noninvasive, this is the most promising tool for neuroimaging research, as it allows us to stimulate brain circuits while monitoring changes in the brain's activity and behavior in humans (Bohning, et al. 1999, Caparelli 2007, Hallett 2000, Hallett 2007, Siebner, et al. 2003). This methodology can help to identify brain networks associated with a specific function, supporting causality for brain-behavior connections, and to assess directly the neural effects of a TMS stimulus across the entire brain. However, the direct interaction between the TMS pulse and the MRI scanners poses a considerable technical challenge; thus, few research groups have implemented this approach successfully (Bestmann, et al. 2003, Bohning, et al. 2003)

TMS and fMRI – Technical issues

The main technical issue in simultaneously implementing TMS and fMRI lies, in safely and correctly, positioning the TMS inside the MRI scanner. When two magnetic fields are generated at the same space they interact and induce a reaction force over the sources that will rotate them to align the source's poles, a phenomenon called the torque reaction. For example, when a magnet is in the presence of an external magnetic field, it experiences a torque that tends to align the magnet's poles with the direction of the magnetic field's lines. Similarly, when a TMS coil generates a time- varying magnetic field inside an MRI scanner, i.e., under another high static magnetic field, a torque reaction will act over the TMS coil (Reitz, et al. 1993). These torque reactions are proportion to the scanner's external magnetic field, and depend on the coil's shape and composition (ferromagnetic or non-ferromagnetic), and current direction inside the TMS coil. For example, in a figure-of-eight MRI-compatible TMS coil, using a biphasic stimulator, that generates electrical currents flowing in the opposite direction (Figure 6), the torque reaction is not considered strong (Bohning, et al.

1998); however, it may be significant if another coil shape, or a monophasic stimulator is used. Therefore, to accurately and safely place the TMS coil on the chosen brain site for magnetic stimulation inside the MRI scanners, each MRI center has customized the coil holders to fulfill their needs according with their experiment set up. Thus, Bestmann and colleagues (2003) attached a plastic holder to the head RF-coil that can be manually adjusted (Bestmann, et al. 2003); the wooden approach has been also used as an MRI compatible TMS coil holder (one example developed at BNL, appears in Figure 7 and another in ref. (Bestmann, et al. 2004). A further approach is the semi- automatic TMS coil positioning/holding system, developed by Bohning and colleagues; it is a compact holder, manually operated with 6 calibrated degrees of freedom and with a software package for transforming the MR images' coordinates to the MRI scanner space coordinates (Bohning, et al. 2003).

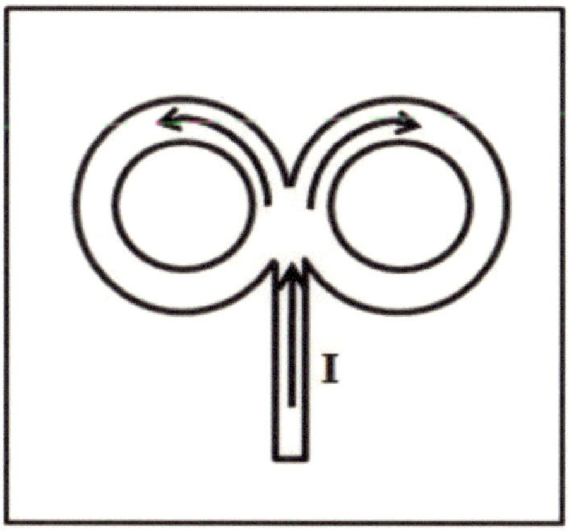

Fig. 6. Figure-of-eight TMS coil with the shown the current directions when used in a biphasic stimulator

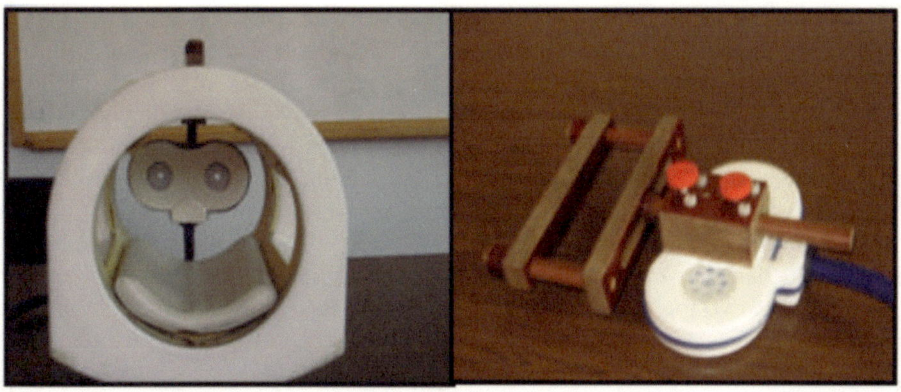

Fig. 7. Picture of the TMS coil holder developed at Brookhaven National Laboratory; left: RF-coil, TMS coil, and coil holder; and, right: TMS coil and coil holder.

The other technical issue associated with this multimodality combination is the interference generated by the TMS coil and the MRI's imaging acquisition process, which was explored by the "pioneers" in using this multimodality technique (Bestmann, et al. 2003). In a magnetic field of 2 Tesla, aliasing and/or susceptibility artifacts might occur, depending on the orientation of the TMS coil and image acquisition, Furthermore, the TMS pulse can interfere with the image acquisition if the interval between the TMS pulse and the first RF excitation pulse is less than about 100 ms. New versions of the MRI-compatible TMS coil minimize the possibility of having aliasing artifacts, while the outcomes of susceptibility artifacts (Figure 8), and the timing between the TMS pulse and image acquisition vary with different magnetic fields.

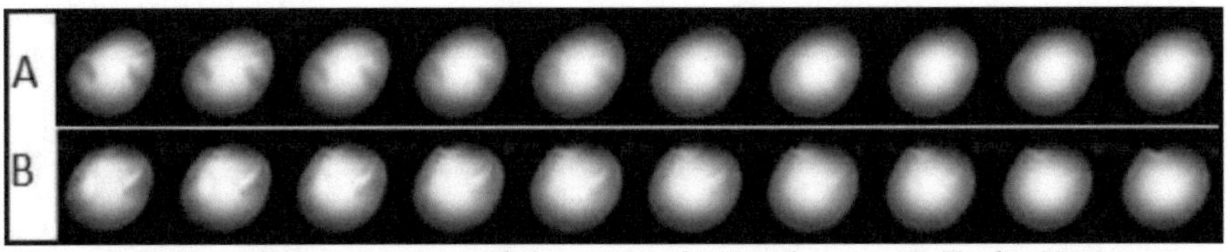

Fig. 8. Round water-phantom coronal images obtained in a 4 Tesla Varian scanner at Brookhaven National Laboratory, without the TMS coil (A), and with the TMS positioned, as shown in figure 7, perpendicular to the image orientation. Local artifacts are observed at the contact point between TMS coil and the phantom (top of fig. B).

Initial applications

The feasibility of simultaneous TMS and fMRI was initially demonstrated in 1.5 Tesla MRI scanners using low frequency TMS protocols (single-pulse TMS or 1 Hz rTMS) and it was considered relatively safe (Bohning, et al. 1998, Bohning, et al. 1999, Bohning, et al. 2000, Bohning, et al. 2000, Bohning, et al. 2003). These researchers used the simultaneous TMS-fMRI technique to evaluate brain activation induced by TMS stimuli of varying intensity applied over the motor cortex region. They directly correlated stimulus intensity and brain activation, but, even though the activated networks generated by different intensities were similar, the areas activated by supra-motor-threshold TMS displayed a bigger BOLD signal than those resulting from sub-motor threshold TMS stimuli. They have also observed some activation in the auditory cortex from the loud noise caused by TMS pulse.

Later studies employed this combination to explore brain activation induced by TMS stimulus given in different brain regions (Nahas, et al. 2001), and with higher rTMS frequencies in higher static magnetic fields, such as 2 Tesla (Baudewig, et al. 2001, Bestmann, et al. 2003) and 3 Tesla MRI scanners (Bestmann, et al. 2004), while also varying the stimulus intensity. These groups verified once more that higher stimulus intensity induces activated areas with a larger cluster size than those activated by a stimulus of lesser intensity. Furthermore, they observed that highfrequency rTMS induces brain activation in a larger network than that induced by a lower rTMs frequency. Thus, in applying a 4 Hz rTMS stimulus at two intensities , supra- and sub-threshold, over the left supplementary motor cortex (M1/S1) in a 2 T MRI scanner, Bestmann and colleagues observed brain activation on the site of stimulation, bilaterally on the right M1/S1, supplementary motor cortex (SMA) and lateral premotor cortex (LPMC) for supra-threshold TMS stimulus. In constrast, there were no significant BOLD-fMRI responses to sub-thresholds stimulations at the stimulus site, but they were evident at distant brain regions, viz, the SMA, LPMC and contralateral M1/S1. (Bestmann, et al. 2003).

Current situation - possibilities and limitations

Existing research results, using the simultaneous combination of TMS and fMRI in different magnetic field intensities, already demonstrated that the technique is feasible and sufficiently safe as a routine research tool in normal volunteers. Its use was extended from the motor cortex to others brain areas, such as the premotor cortex (Bestmann, et al. 2005), frontal-eyes-field (Ruff, et al. 2006), parietal cortex (Ruff, et al. 2008) and occipital area (Caparelli, et al. 2010). The published studies show that this multimodality technique provides the ability to monitor BOLD response while allowing the precise selection of the anatomic- and functional-targets through TMS stimulus, so affording a robust tool for investigating the connection between the TMS action in the cortex areas, and the subsequent BOLD response in subcortical regions.

Nevertheless, although the feasibility of this combined technique is well established, and its several advantages for neuroimaging research enumerated, simultaneous TMS and MRI still technically challenges most research centers. Accordingly, more technical development is needed to reduce the size and shape of the TMS coils so they can fit inside the current multichannel receivers RF-coils. Further, since current MRI compatible TMS coil shape restrict the areas of stimulation to the cortical region, progress is much needed to ensure we can apply a deep TMS stimulus and simultaneously measure the brain's response.

5. References

Amassian, V. E., Cracco, R. Q., Maccabee, P. J., Cracco, J. B., Rudell, A. and Eberle, L. (1989) Suppression of visual perception by magnetic coil stimulation of human occipital cortex. Electroencephalography and clinical neurophysiology, 74, 6, (11-12/1989), 458-462, 0013-4694 (P)

Anand, S. and Hotson, J. (2002) Transcranial magnetic stimulation: neurophysiological applications and safety. Brain and Cognition, 50, 3, (12/2002), 366-386, 0278-2626 (P)

Bandettini, P. A., Wong, E. C., Hinks, R. S., Tikofky, R. S. and Hyde, J. S. (1992) Time course EPI of human brain function during task activation. Magnetic Resonance Medicine, 25, 2, (06/1992), 390-397, 0740-3194 (P)

Barker, A. T., Jalinous, R. and Freeston, I. L. (1985) Non-invasive magnetic stimulation of human motor cortex. Lancet, 1, 8437, (05/1995), 1106-1107, 0140-6736 (P)

Bastings, E. P., Gage, H. D., Greenberg, J. P., Hammond, G., Hernandez, L., Santago, P., Hamilton, C. A., Moody, D. M., Singh, K. D., Ricci, P. E., Pons, T. P. and Good, D. C. (1998) Co-registration of cortical magnetic stimulation and functional magnetic resonance imaging. Neuroreport, 9, 9, (06/1998), 1941-1946, 0959-4965 (P)

Baudewig, J., Siebner, H. R., Bestmann, S., Tergau, F., Tings, T., Paulus, W. and Frahm, J. (2001) Functional MRI of cortical activations induced by transcranial magnetic stimulation (TMS). Neuroreport., 12, 16, (11/2001), 3543-48, 0959-4965 (P)

Beckers, G. and Zeki, S. (1995) The consequences of inactivating areas V1 and V5 on visual motion perception. Brain, 118, Pt 1, (02/1995), 49-60, 0006-8950 (P)

Ben-Shachar, D., Belmaker, R. H., Grisaru, N. and Klein, E. (1997) Transcranial magnetic stimulation induces alterations in brain monoamines. Journal of Neural Transmission, 104, 2-3, (02/1997), 191-197, 0300-9564 (P)

Berardelli, A., Inghilleri, M., Cruccu, G., Mercuri, B. and Manfredi, M. (1991) Electrical and magnetic transcranial stimulation in patients with corticospinal damage due to stroke or motor neurone disease. Electroencephalography and clinical neurophysiology, 81, 5, (10/1991), 389-396, 0013-4694 (P)

Bestmann, S., Baudewig, J. and Frahm, J. (2003) On the Synchronization of Transcranial Magnetic Stimulation and Functional Echo-Planar Imaging. Journal of Magnetic Resonance Imaging, 17, 3, (03/2003), 309-316, 1053-1807 (P)

Bestmann, S., Baudewig, J., Siebner, H. R., Rothwell, J. C. and Frahm, J. (2003) Subthreshold high-frequency TMS of human primary motor cortex modulates interconnected frontal motor areas as detected by interleaved fMRI-TMS. Neuroimage, 20, 3, (11/2003), 1685-96, 1053-8119 (P)

Bestmann, S., Baudewig, J., Siebner, H. R., Rothwell, J. C. and Frahm, J. (2004) Functional MRI of the immediate impact of transcranial magnetic stimulation on cortical and subcortical motor circuits. The European journal of neuroscience, 19, 7, (04/2004), 1950-62, 0953-816X (P)

Bestmann, S., Baudewig, J., Siebner, H. R., Rothwell, J. C. and Frahm, J. (2005) BOLD MRI responses to repetitive TMS over human dorsal premotor cortex. Neuroimage, 28, 1, (10/2005), 22-9, 1053-8119 (P)

Bickford, R. G. and Fremming, B. D. (1965). Neuronal stimulation by pulsed magnetic fields in animals and man. Digest of the 6th International Conference in Medical Electronics and Biological Engineering.p.112, IFMBE.

Bohning, D. E., Shastri, A., Nahas, Z., Lorberbaum, J. P., Andersen, S. W., Dannels, W. R., Haxthausen, E. U., Vincent, D. J. and George, M. S. (1998) Echoplanar BOLD fMRI of brain activation induced by concurrent transcranial magnetic stimulation. Investigative radiology, 33, 6, (06/1998), 336-40, 0020-9996 (P)

Bohning, D. E., Shastri, A., McConnell, K. A., Nahas, Z., Lorberbaum, J. P., Roberts, D. R., Teneback, C., Vincent, D. J. and George, M. S. (1999) A combined TMS/fMRI study of intensity-dependent TMS over motor cortex. Biological Psychiatry, 45, 4, (02/1999), 385-94, 0006-3223 (P)

Bohning, D. E., Shastri, A., McGavin, L., McConnell, K. A., Nahas, Z., Lorberbaum, J. P., Roberts, D. R. and George, M. S. (2000) Motor cortex brain activity induced by 1-Hz transcranial magnetic stimulation is similar in location and level to that for volitional movement. Investigative radiology, 35, 11, (11/2000), 676-83, 0020-9996 (P)

Bohning, D. E., Shastri, A., Wassermann, E. M., Ziemann, U., Lorberbaum, J. P., Nahas, Z., Lomarev, M. P. and George, M. S. (2000) BOLD-f MRI response to single-pulse transcranial magnetic stimulation (TMS). Journal of Magnetic Resonance Imaging, 11, 6, (06/2000), 569-574, 1053-1807 (P)

Bohning, D. E., Denslow, S., Bohning, P. A., Walker, J. A. and George, M. S. (2003) A TMS coil positioning/holding system for MR image-guided TMS interleaved with fMRI. Clinical neurophysiology, 114, 11, (11/2003), 2210-2219, 1388-2457 (P)

Bohning, D. E., Shastri, A., Lomarev, M. P., Lorberbaum, J. P., Nahas, Z. and George, M. S. (2003) BOLD-fMRI response vs. transcranial magnetic stimulation (TMS) pulse-train length: testing for linearity. Journal of magnetic resonance imaging, 17, 3, (03/2003), 279-90, 1053-1807 (P)

Boroojerdi, B., Foltys, H., Krings, T., Spetzger, U., Thron, A. and Topper, R. (1999) Localization of the motor hand area using transcranial magnetic stimulation and functional magnetic resonance imaging. Clinical neurophysiology, 110, 4, (04/1999), 699-704, 1388-2457 (P)

Boroojerdi, B., Bushara, K. O., Corwell, B., Immisch, I., Battaglia, F., Muellbacher, W. and Cohen, L. G. (2000) Enhanced excitability of the human visual cortex induced by short-term light deprivation. Cerebral cortex, 10, 5, (05/2000), 529-534, 1047-3211 (P)

Bridgers, S. L. (1991) The safety of transcranial magnetic stimulation reconsidered: evidence regarding cognitive and other cerebral effects. Electroencephalography and clinical neurophysiology. Supplement, 43, 170-179, 0424-8155 (P)

Burt, T., Lisanby, S. H. and Sackeim, H. A. (2002) Neuropsychiatric applications of transcranial magnetic stimulation: a meta analysis. The International Journal of Neuropsychopharmacology, 5, 1, (3/2002), 5,1, 73-103, 1461-1457 (P)

Caparelli, E. C., Tomasi, D., Arnold, S., Chang, L. and Ernst, T. (2003) k-Space based summary motion detection for functional magnetic resonance imaging. NeuroImage, 20, (10/2003) 1411-1418, 1053-8119 (P)

Caparelli, E. C. (2007) TMS&fMRI - A new neuroimaging combinational tool to study brain function. Current Medical Imaging Reviews, 3, 2, 109-115, 1573-4056 (P)

Caparelli, E. C., Backus, W., Telang, F., Wang, G.-J., Maloney, T., Goldstein, R. Z., Anschel, D. and Henn, F. (2010) Simultaneous TMS-fMRI of the visual cortex reveals functional network, even in absence of phosphene sensation. The Open Neuroimaging Journal, (In Press), 1874-4400 (E)

Caramia, M. D., Iani, C. and Bernardi, G. (1996) Cerebral plasticity after stroke as revealed by ipsilateral responses to magnetic stimulation. Neuroreport, 7, 11, (7/1996),1756-1760, 0959-4965 (P)

Cavin, I., Glover, P., Bowtell, R. and Gowland, P. (2007) Thresholds for Perceiving Metallic Taste at High Magnetic Field. Journal Of Magnetic Resonance Imaging, 26, 5, (11/2007), 1357-1361, 1053-1807 (P)

Chakeres, D. W. and de Vocht, F. (2005) Static magnetic field effects on human subjects related to magnetic resonance imaging systems. Progress in Biophysics and Molecular Biology, 87, 2-3, (02-04/2005), 255-265, 0079-6107 (P)

Chen, R., Tam, A., Bütefisch, C., Corwell, B., Ziemann, U., Rothwell, J. C. and Cohen, L. G. (1998) Intracortical inhibition and facilitation in different representations of the human motor cortex. Journal of Neurophysiology, 80, 6, (12/1998), 2870-2881, 0022-3077 (P)

Chokroverty, S., Hening, W., Wright, D., Walczak, T., Goldberg, J., Burger, R., Belsh, J., Patel, B., Flynn, D., Shah, S. and et, a. (1995) Magnetic brain stimulation: safety studies. Electroencephalography and clinical neurophysiology, 97, 1, (2, 1995), 36-42, 0013-4694 (P)

Cox, R. W. (1996) AFNI: Software for analysis and visualization of functional magnetic resonance neuroimages. Computers and Biomedical Research, 29, 3, (6/1996), 162-173,0010-4809 (P)

Cracco, R. Q., Amassian, V. E., Maccabee, P. J. and Cracco, J. B. (1989) Comparison of human transcallosal responses evoked by magnetic coil and electrical stimulation. Electroencephalography and clinical neurophysiology, 74, 6, (11-12/1989), 417-424, 0013-4694 (P)

Daskalakis, Z. J., Levinson, A. J. and Fitzgerald, P. B. (2008) Repetitive transcranial magnetic stimulation for major depressive disorder: a review. Canadian Journal of Psychiatry, 53, 9, (9/2008), 555-566, 0706-7437 (P)

Devlin, J. T., Matthews, P. M. and Rushworth, M. F. (2003) Semantic processing in the left inferior prefrontal cortex: a combined functional magnetic resonance imaging and transcranial magnetic stimulation study. Journal of cognitive neuroscience, 15, 1, (1/2003), 71-84, 0898-929X (P)

Epstein, C. M., Schwartzberg, D. G., Davey, K. R. and Sudderth, D. B. (1990) Localizing the site of magnetic brain stimulation in humans. Neurology, 40, 4, (4/1990), 666-670, 0028-3878 (P)

Flitman, S. S., Grafman, J., Wassermann, E. M., Cooper, V., O'Grady, J., Pascual-Leone, A. and Hallett, M. (1998) Linguistic processing during repetitive transcranial magnetic stimulation. Neurology, 50, 1, (1/1998), 175-181,0028-3878 (P)

Fox, P. T. and Raichle, M. E. (1985) Stimulus rate determines regional brain blood flow in striate cortex. Annals of Neurology, 17, 3, (3/1985), 303-305, 0364-5134 (P)

Fregni, F., Ono, C. R., Santos, C. M., Bermpohl, F., Buchpiguel, C., Barbosa, E. R., Marcolin, M. A., Pascual-Leone, A. and Valente, K. D. (2006) Effects of antidepressant treatment with rTMS and fluoxetine on brain perfusion in PD. Neurology, 66, 11, (6/2006), 1629-1637, 0028-3878 (P)

Friston, K., Harrison, L. and Penny, W. (2003) Dynamic causal modelling. Neuroimage, 19, 4, (8/2003), 1273-1302,1053-8119 (P)

Friston, K. J. (1996). Statistical parametric mapping and other analyses of functional imaging data. Brain mapping: The methods. A. W. Toga and J. C. Mazziotta, 363-386, Academic Press, San Diego.

Gati, J. S., Menon, R. S., Ugurbil, K. and Rutt, B. K. (1997) Experimental determination of the BOLD field strength dependence in vessels and tissue. Magnetic Resonance in Medicine, 38, 296-302, (8/1997), 0740-3194 (P)

George, M. S., Wassermann, E. M., Williams, W. A., Callahan, A., Ketter, T. A., Basser, P., Hallett, M. and Post, R. M. (1995) Daily repetitive transcranial magnetic stimulation (rTMS) improves mood in depression. Neuroreport, 6, 14, (10/1995),1853-1856, 0959-4965 (P)

George, M. S., Wassermann, E. M., Kimbrell, T. A., Little, J. T., Williams, W. E., Danielson, A. L., Greenberg, B. D., Hallett, M. and Post, R. M. (1997) Mood improvement following daily left prefrontal repetitive transcranial magnetic stimulation in patients with depression: a placebo-controlled crossover trial. The American journal of psychiatry, 154, 2, (12/1997), 1752-1756, 0002-953X (P)

Glover, P., Cavin, I., Qian, W., Bowtell, R. and Gowland, P. (2007) Magnetic-field-induced vertigo: a theoretical and experimental investigation. Bioelectromagnetics., 28, 5, (07/2007), 349-361, 0197-8462 (P)

Glover, P. M. (2009) Interaction of MRI field gradients with the human body. Physics in Medicine and Biology, 54, 21, (11/2009), R99-R115, 0031-9155 (P)

Griskova, I., Hoppner, J., Ruksenas, O. and Dapsys, K. (2006) Transcranial magnetic stimulation: the method and application. Medicina (Kaunas, Lithuania), 42, 10, 798-804, 1010-660X (P)

Hada, Y., Abo, M., Kaminaga, T. and Mikami, M. (2006) Detection of cerebral blood flow changes during repetitive transcranial magnetic stimulation by recording hemoglobin in the brain cortex, just beneath the stimulation coil, with near-infrared spectroscopy. Neuroimage, 32, 3, (9/2006), 1226-1230, 1053-8119 (P)

Hallett, M. (2000) Transcranial magnetic stimulation and the human brain. Nature, 406, 6792, (7/2000) ,147-150, 0028-0836 (P)

Hallett, M. (2007) Transcranial magnetic stimulation: a primer. Neuron, 55, 2, (7/2007) 187-199, 0896-6273 (P)

Hamdy, S., Aziz, Q., Rothwell, J. C., Singh, K. D., Barlow, J., Hughes, D. G., Tallis, R. C. and Thompson, D. G. (1996) The cortical topography of human swallowing musculature in health and disease. Nature medicine, 2, 11, (11/1996), 1217-1224, 1078-8956 (P)

Hinke, R. M., Hu, X., Stillman, A. E., Kim, S. G., Merkle, H., Salmi, R. and Ugurbil, K. (1993) Functional magnetic resonance imaging of Broca's area during internal speech. Neuroreport, 4, 6, (6/1993), 675-678, 0959-4965 (P)

Jackson, J. D. (1965). Classical Electrodynamics. New York, John Wiley and Sons.

Jalinouz, R. (1998). Guide for Magnetic Stimulation, Magstim: http://www.magstim.com/downloads/.

Kandler, R. (1990) Safety of transcranial magnetic stimulation. Lancet, 335, 8687, (2/1990), 469-470, 0140-6736 (P)

Keck, M. E., Sillaber, I., Ebner, K., Welt, T., Toschi, N., Kaehler, S. T., Singewald, N., Philippu, A., Elbel, G. K., Wotjak, C. T., Holsboer, F., Landgraf, R. and Engelmann, M. (2000) Acute transcranial magnetic stimulation of frontal brain regions selectively modulates the release of vasopressin, biogenic amines and amino acids in the rat brain. The European journal of neuroscience, 12, 10, (10/2000), 3713-3720, 0953-816X (P)

Keck, M. E., Welt, T., Post, A., Muller, M. B., Toschi, N., Wigger, A., Landgraf, R., Holsboer, F. and Engelmann, M. (2001) Neuroendocrine and behavioral effects of repetitive transcranial magnetic stimulation in a psychopathological animal model are suggestive of antidepressant-like effects. Neuropsychopharmacology, 24, 4, (4/2001), (337-349, 0893-133X (P)

Keck, M. E., Welt, T., Muller, M. B., Erhardt, A., Ohl, F., Toschi, N., Holsboer, F. and Sillaber, I. (2002) Repetitive transcranial magnetic stimulation increases the release of dopamine in the mesolimbic and mesostriatal system. Neuropharmacology, 43, 1, (7/2002), 101-109, 0028-3908 (P)

Kew, J. J., Ridding, M. C., Rothwell, J. C., Passingham, R. E., Leigh, P. N., Sooriakumaran, S., Frackowiak, R. S. and Brooks, D. J. (1994) Reorganization of cortical blood flow and transcranial magnetic stimulation maps in human subjects after upper limb amputation. Journal of neurophysiology, 72, 5, (11/1994), 2517-2524, 0022-3077 (P)

Kim, S. G., Ashe, J. and Hendrich, K. (1993) Functional magnetic resonance imaging of motor cortex: hemispheric asymmetry and handedness. Science, 261, 5121, (7/1993), 615-617, 0193-4511 (P)

Kole, M. H., Fuchs, E., Ziemann, U., Paulus, W. and Ebert, U. (1999) Changes in 5-HT1A and NMDA binding sites by a single rapid transcranial magnetic stimulation procedure in rats. Brain Research, 826, 2, (5/1999), (309-312, 0006-8993 (P)

Kujirai, T., Caramia, M. D., Rothwell, J. C., Day, B. L., Thompson, P. D., Ferbert, A., Wroe, S., Asselman, P. and Marsden, C. D. (1993) Corticocortical inhibition in human motor cortex. The Journal of physiology, 471, (11/1993), 501-519, 0022-3751 (P)

Lisanby, S. H., Luber, B., Perera, T. and Sackeim, H. A. (2000) Transcranial magnetic stimulation: applications in basic neuroscience and neuropsychopharmacology. The international journal of neuropsychopharmacology, 3, 3, (9/2000), 259-273, 1461-1457 (P)

Little, J. T., Kimbrell, T. A., Wassermann, E. M., Grafman, J., Figueras, S., Dunn, R. T., Danielson, A., Repella, J., Huggins, T., George, M. S. and Post, R. M. (2000) Cognitive effects of 1- and 20-hertz repetitive transcranial magnetic stimulation in depression: preliminary report. Neuropsychiatry, neuropsychology, and behavioral neurology., 13, 2, (4/2000), 119-124, 0894-878X (P)

Meyer, B. U., Roricht, S. and Woiciechowsky, C. (1998) Topography of fibers in the human corpus callosum mediating interhemispheric inhibition between the motor cortices. Annals of neurology, 43, 3, (3/1998), 360-369, 0364-5134 (P)

Miller, M. B., Fendrich, R., Eliassen, J. C., Demirel, S. and Gazzaniga, M. S. (1996) Transcranial magnetic stimulation: delays in visual suppression due to luminance changes. Neuroreport, 7, 11, (07/1996), 1740-1744, 0959-4965 (P)

Moelker, A. and Pattynama, P. (2003) Acoustic noise concerns in functional magnetic resonance imaging. Human Brain Mapping, 20, 3, (11/2003), 123-141, 1065-9471 (P)

Muri, R. M., Rivaud, S., Vermersch, A. I., Leger, J. M. and Pierrot-Deseilligny, C. (1995) Effects of transcranial magnetic stimulation over the region of the supplementary motor area during sequences of memory-guided saccades. Experimental brain research, 104, 1, 163-166, 0014-4819 (P)

Nahas, Z., Lomarev, M., Roberts, D. R., Shastri, A., Lorberbaum, J. P., Teneback, C., McConnell, K., Vincent, D. J., Li, X., George, M. S. and Bohning, D. E. (2001) Unilateral left prefrontal transcranial magnetic stimulation (TMS) produces intensity-dependent bilateral effects as measured by interleaved BOLD fMRI. Biological psychiatry, 50, 9, (11/2001), 712-720, 0006-3223 (P)

Ogawa, S., Lee, T. M., Kay, A. R. and Tank, D. W. (1990). Brain magnetic resonance imaging with contrast dependent on blood oxygenation. Proceedings of the National Academy of Sciences of the United States of America, 87.9868-9872.

Ogawa, S., Tank, D. W., Menon, R. S., Ellerman, J. M., Kim, S. G., Merkle, H. and Ugurbil, K. (1992). Intrinsic signal changes accompanying sensory stimulation: Functional brain mapping with magnetic resonance imaging. Proceedings of the National Academy of Sciences of the United States of America, 89.5951-5955.

Oh, S., Webb, A. G., Neuberger, T., Park, B. and Collins, C. M. (2010) Experimental and numerical assessment of MRI-induced temperature change and SAR distributions in phantoms and in vivo. Magnetic Resonance in Medicine, 63, 1, (01/2010), 218-223, 1347-3182 (P)

Okada, T., Yamada, H., Ito, H., Yonekura, Y. and Sadato, N. (2005) Magnetic field strength increase yields significantly greater contrast-to-noise ratio increase: Measured using BOLD contrast in the primary visual area. Academic Radiology, 12, 2, (2/2005), 142-147, 1076-6332 (P)

Pascual-Leone, A., Grafman, J. and Hallett, M. (1994) Modulation of cortical motor output maps during development of implicit and explicit knowledge. Science, 263, 5151, (3/1994), 1287-1289, 0193-4511 (P)

Pascual-Leone, A., Valls-Sole, J., Brasil-Neto, J. P., Cammarota, A., Grafman, J. and Hallett, M. (1994) Akinesia in Parkinson's disease. II. Effects of subthreshold repetitive transcranial motor cortex stimulation. Neurology, 44, 5, (5/1994), 892-898, 0028-3878 (P)

Pascual-Leone, A., Rubio, B., Pallardo, F. and Catala, M. D. (1996) Rapid-rate transcranial magnetic stimulation of left dorsolateral prefrontal cortex in drug-resistant depression. Lancet, 348, 9022, (7/1996), 233-237, 0140-6736 (P)

Pauling, L. and Coryell, C. D. (1936) The Magnetic Properties and Structure of Hemoglobin, Oxyhemoglobin and Carbonmonoxyhemoglobin. Proceedings of the National Academy of Sciences of the United States of America, 22, 4, (03/1936), 210-216, 0027-8424 (P)

Paus, T., Jech, R., Thompson, C. J., Comeau, R., Peters, T. and Evans, A. C. (1997) Transcranial magnetic stimulation during positron emission tomography: a new method for studying connectivity of the human cerebral cortex. The Journal of neuroscience, 17, 9, (5/1997), 3178-84, 0270-6474 (P)

Paus, T. and Wolforth, M. (1998) Transcranial magnetic stimulation during PET: reaching and verifying the target site. Human brain mapping, 6, 5-6, 399-402, 1065-9471 (P)

Pernet, C., Schyns, P. G. and Demonet, J. F. (2007) Specific, selective or preferential: comments on category specificity in neuroimaging. Neuroimage, 35, 3, (4/2007), 991-997, 1053-8119 (P)

Polson, M. J., Barker, A. T. and Freeston, I. L. (1982) Stimulation of nerve trunks with time-varying magnetic fields. Medical & Biological Engineering & Computing, 20, 2, (3/1982), 243-244, 0140-0118 (P)

Post, A. and Keck, M. E. (2001) Transcranial magnetic stimulation as a therapeutic tool in psychiatry: what do we know about the neurobiological mechanisms? Journal of Psychiatric Research, 35, 4, (7-8/2001), 193-215, 0022-3956 (P)

Pruessmann, K., Weiger, M., Scheidegger, M. and Boesiger, P. (1999) SENSE: sensitivity encoding for fast MRI. Magnetic Resonance in Medicine, 42, 5, (11/1999), 952-962, 0740-3194 (P)

Puri, B. K., Davey, N. J., Ellaway, P. H. and Lewis, S. W. (1996) An investigation of motor function in schizophrenia using transcranial magnetic stimulation of the motor cortex. The British journal of psychiatry, 169, 6, (12/1996), 690-695, 0007-1250 (P)

Raichle, M. E. and Mintun, M. A. (2006) Brain work and brain imaging. Annual review of neuroscience, 29, (7/2006), 449-476, 0147-006X (P)

Rapisarda, G., Bastings, E., de Noordhout, A. M., Pennisi, G. and Delwaide, P. J. (1996) Can motor recovery in stroke patients be predicted by early transcranial magnetic stimulation? Stroke, 27, 12, (12/1996), 2191-2196, 0147-006X (P)

Reitz, J. R., Milford, F. J. and Christy, R. W. (1993). Foundations of Electromagnetic Theory. New York, Addison-Wesley Publishing Company, Inc.

Roberts, D. R., Vincent, D. J., Speer, A. M., Bohning, D. E., Cure, J., Young, J. and George, M. S. (1997) Multi-modality mapping of motor cortex: comparing echoplanar BOLD fMRI and transcranial magnetic stimulation. Short communication. Journal of neural transmission, 104, 8-9, 833-843, 0300-9564 (P)

Rossi, S., Hallett, M., Rossini, P. M. and Pascual-Leone, A. (2009) Safety, ethical considerations, and application guidelines for the use of transcranial magnetic stimulation in clinical practice and research. Clinical neurophysiology 20, 12, (12/2009), 2008-2039, 1388-2457 (P)

Rostrup, E., Larsson, H. B., Toft, P. B., Garde, K., Ring, P. B. and Henriksen, O. (1996) Susceptibility contrast imaging of CO2-induced changes in the blood volume of the human brain. Acta Radiologica, 37, 5, (9/1996), 813-822, 0001-6926 (P)

Roy, C. S. and Sherrington, C. S. (1890) On the Regulation of the Blood-supply of the Brain. The Journal of physiology, 11, 1-2, (1/1890), 85-158.17, 0022-3751 (P)

Rudiak, D. and Marg, E. (1994) Finding the depth of magnetic brain stimulation: a re-evaluation. Electroencephalography and Clinical Neurophysiology, 93, 5, (10/1994), 358-371, 0013-4694 (P)

Ruff, C. C., Blankenburg, F., Bjoertomt, O., Bestmann, S., Freeman, E., Haynes, J. D., Rees, G., Josephs, O., Deichmann, R. and Driver, J. (2006) Concurrent TMS-fMRI and psychophysics reveal frontal influences on human retinotopic visual cortex. Current biology, 16, 15, (8/2006), 1479-88, 0960-9822 (P)

Ruff, C. C., Bestmann, S., Blankenburg, F., Bjoertomt, O., Josephs, O., Weiskopf, N., Deichmann, R. and Driver, J. (2008) Distinct causal influences of parietal versus frontal areas on human visual cortex: evidence from concurrent TMS-fMRI. Cerebral cortex 18, 4, (4/2008), 817-27, 1047-3211 (P)

Sack, A. T. and Linden, D. E. (2003) Combining transcranial magnetic stimulation and functional imaging in cognitive brain research: possibilities and limitations. Brain research. Brain research reviews, 43, 1, (9,2003), 41-56.

Sack, A. T. (2006) Transcranial magnetic stimulation, causal structure-function mapping and networks of functional relevance. Current Opinion in Neurobiology, 16, 5, (10/2006), 593-599, 0959-4388 (P)

Schlaepfer, T. E. and Kosel, M. (2004). Transcranial magnetic stimulation in depression. Brain stimulation in psychiatric treatment. S. H. Lisanby, 1-22, American Psychiatric Publishing, Washington DC.

Schutter, D. J. and van Honk, J. (2006) An electrophysiological link between the cerebellum, cognition and emotion: Frontal theta EEG activity to single-pulse cerebellar TMS. Neuroimage, 33, 4, (12/2006), 1227-1231, 1053-8119 (P)

Siebner, H. R., Lee, L. and Bestmann, S. (2003) Interleaving TMS with functional MRI: now that it is technically feasible how should it be used? Clinical neurophysiology, 114, 11, (11/2003), 1997-99, 1388-2457 (P)

Smith, S. M., Jenkinson, M., Woolrich, M. W., Beckmann, C. F., Behrens, T. E., Johansen-Berg, H., Bannister, P. R., De Luca, M., Drobnjak, I., Flitney, D. E., Niazy, R. K., Saunders, J., Vickers, J., Zhang, Y., De Stefano, N., Brady, J. M. and Matthews, P. M. (2004) Advances in functional and structural MR image analysis and implementation as FSL. Neuroimage, 23, Suppl1, S208-S219, 1053-8119 (P)

Song, A. W., Harshbarger, T., Li, T., Kim, K. H., Ugurbil, K., Mori, S. and Kim, D. S. (2003) Functional activation using apparent diffusion coefficient-dependent contrast allows better spatial localization to the neuronal activity: evidence using diffusion tensor imaging and fiber tracking. Neuroimage, 20, 2, (10/2003), 955-961, 1053-8119 (P)

Speer, A. M., Kimbrell, T. A., Wassermann, E. M., D Repella, J., Willis, M. W., Herscovitch, P. and Post, R. M. (2000) Opposite effects of high and low frequency rTMS on regional brain activity in depressed patients. Biological psychiatry, 48, 12, (12/2000), 1133-1141, 0006-3223 (P)

Stecco, A., Saponaro, A. and Carriero, A. (2007) Patient safety issues in magnetic resonance imaging: state of the art. La Radiologia medica, 112, 4, (06/2007), 491-508, 0033-8362 (P)

Stewart, L. M., Walsh, V. and Rothwell, J. C. (2001) Motor and phosphene thresholds: a transcranial magnetic stimulation correlation study. Neuropsychologia, 39, 4, 415-419, 0028-3932 (P)

Strafella, A. P., Paus, T., Barrett, J. and Dagher, A. (2001) Repetitive transcranial magnetic stimulation of the human prefrontal cortex induces dopamine release in the caudate nucleus. The Journal of neuroscience, 21, 15, (8/2001), RC157, 0270-6474 (P)

Tada, H., Rappaport, J., Lashgari, M., Amini, S., Wong-Staal, F. and Khalili, K. (1990) Trans-activation of the JC virus late promoter by the tat protein to type 1 human immunodeficiency virus in glial cells. Proceedings of the National Academy of Sciences, 87, 9,(5/1990), 3479-3483, 0027-8424 (P)

Thompson, S. P. (1910). A physiological effect of an alternating magnetic field. Proc. Royal Society (Biol.), 82.396-398.

Thut, G., Northoff, G., Ives, J. R., Kamitani, Y., Pfennig, A., Kampmann, F., Schomer, D. L. and Pascual-Leone, A. (2003) Effects of single-pulse transcranial magnetic stimulation (TMS) on functional brain activity: a combined event-related TMS and evoked potential study. Clinical neurophysiology, 114, 11, (11/2003), 2071-2080, 1388-2457 (P)

Tokimura, H., Tokimura, Y., Oliviero, A., Asakura, T. and Rothwell, J. C. (1996) Speech-induced changes in corticospinal excitability. Annals of neurology, 40, 4, (10/1996), 628-634, 0364-5134 (P)

Tomasi, D., Chang, L., Caparelli, E. C. and Ernst, T. (2007) Different activation patterns for working memory load and visual attention load. Brain research, 1132, 1, (2/2007), 158-165, 0006-8993 (P)

Triggs, W. J., McCoy, K. J., Greer, R., Rossi, F., Bowers, D., Kortenkamp, S., Nadeau, S., E, Heilman, K., M and Goodman, W. K. (1999) Effects of left frontal transcranial magnetic stimulation on depressed mood, cognition, and corticomotor threshold. Biological psychiatry, 45, 11, (6/1999), 1440-1446, 0006-3223 (P)

van der Zwaag, W., Francis, S., Head, K., Peters, A., Gowland, P., Morris, P. and Bowtell, R. (2009) fMRI at 1.5, 3 and 7 T: characterising BOLD signal changes. Neuroimage, 47, 4, (10/2009), 1425-1434, 1053-8119 (P)

Wagle, W. A. and Smith, M. (2000) Tattoo-induced skin burn during MR imaging. AJR. American journal of roentgenology, 174, 6, (06/2000), 1795, 0361-803X (P)

Walsh, V. and Cowey, A. (1998) Magnetic stimulation studies of visual cognition. Trends in Cognitive Sciences, 2, 3,(3/1998), 103-110, 1364-6613 (P)

Wassermann, E. M. (1998) Risk and safety of repetitive transcranial magnetic stimulation: report and suggested guidelines from the International Workshop on the Safety of Repetitive Transcranial Magnetic Stimulation, June 5-7, 1996. Electroencephalography and Clinical Neurophysiology, 108, 1, (1/1998), 1-16, 0013-4694 (P)

Wassermann, E. M. and Lisanby, S. H. (2001) Therapeutic application of repetitive transcranial magnetic stimulation: a review. Clinical neurophysiology : official journal of the International Federation of Clinical Neurophysiology, 112, 8, (8/2001, 1367-1377, 1388-2457 (P)

Werhahn, K. J., Lieber, J., Classen, J. and Noachtar, S. (2000) Motor cortex excitability in patients with focal epilepsy. Epilepsy research, 41, 2, (9/2000), 179-189, 0920-1211 (P)

Ziemann, U., Lonnecker, S., Steinhoff, B. J. and Paulus, W. (1996) Effects of antiepileptic drugs on motor cortex excitability in humans: a transcranial magnetic stimulation study. Annals of neurology, 40, 3, (9/1996), 367-378, 0364-5134 (P)

3

Modulation of emotional faces processing and its implication for depression and anxiety

Cristina Marta Del-Ben and Frederico Guilherme Graeff
Division of Psychiatry, Faculty of Medicine of Ribeirão Preto, University of São Paulo
Brazil

1. Introduction

The recognition of environmental information with emotional valence is crucial for the adjustment and social functioning. Since Darwin (1872), facial expressions of basic emotions have been considered as a fundamental component of the processing of emotions and various studies have provided evidence of a dissociable although interconnected involvement of different neural substrates in the emotional processing. Happiness, sadness, anger, fear and disgust are considered as basic emotions. Although with some controversies, surprise is also considered as a basic emotion.

In spite of some contrary positions (e.g. Russell, 1994) facial expressions of basic emotions have been considered as universal, i.e., identified in a similar way in different cultures, whether they are literate or preliterate (Andrew, 1963; Ekman et al., 1969), as originally proposed by Charles Darwin. The studies carried out by Paul Ekman and his colleagues led to the development of a database of photographs of actors and actresses expressing basic emotions, called Pictures of Facial Affect (Ekman & Friesen, 1976), which has been widely used in different paradigms, such as emotional processing and aversive conditioning and, more recently, psychological paradigms of activation associated with functional neuroimaging. Other sets of images with facial expressions (Gur et al., 2002) have also been used.

The facial musculature is complex, diverse and highly specialized. From an evolutionary perspective, the proliferation and diversification of the facial muscles coincide with the development of language and the period of rapid increase in hominid brain size, when they left the rain forest to live on the savannah. Life in groups led gains to secure food through hunting, and safety from predators. On the other hand, guarantee the survival and breeding in large groups required capacity to recognize emotions of other members of the social organization and, therefore, predict their behavior. If the social cues are important components in this new social organization, the ability to identify and translate these signals must have evolved in parallel with the development of the ability to express and manage, at least partially, the facial expressions. Therefore, humans would not be able to communicate emotional signs, but also to decode them quickly and efficiently (Öhman, 2002).

Our innate ability of decoding emotional signs communicated by our peers can be affected by several conditions, such emotional state, personality traits, diagnosis of mental disorders, drug manipulation, among others. In this chapter we will review results about emotional face processing, obtained through different techniques that can bring some information about the pathophysiology of anxiety and mood disorders.

2. Neural substrates of emotional faces processing

The advance of neuroimaging techniques has provided substantial data for the understanding of the neurobiology of the emotional processing in humans. Several paradigms of psychological activation have been examined by magnetic resonance imaging (fMRI) and positron emission tomography (PET) in order to evaluate specific components of the processing of emotions, such as the conscious or unconscious identification perception of basic emotions, fear conditioning, reward and punishment, among others. Studies of fMRI, applying psychological activation paradigms aimed at verifying the neural responses of healthy volunteers to facial expressions of basic emotions, suggest the activation of specific neural substrates for different emotional expressions.

The face perception in humans is mediated by a neuronal system consisted by multiple and bilateral regions (Haxby et al., 2002). This system has a hierarchical organization, initially composed of a system of visual processing of the face, made up of three distinct regions. The first of these regions is the inferior occipital gyrus that captures the general features of the face perception. This region connects to two other regions, the superior temporal sulcus and the fusiform gyrus. The superior temporal sulcus assesses changing aspects of the face, as the perception of gaze direction of the face and mouth movements. The lateral fusiform gyrus analyzes the invariant aspects of the face, giving the unique identity of each face. This system of visual analysis of the face sends links to an extensive neuronal plot with different cognitive functions that can act in accordance with the visual analysis system to give meaning to the faces. The superior temporal sulcus connects with the intraparietal sulcus, responsible for analyzing the spatial direction, related to head movement and direction of the eyes, and the auditory cortex responsible for processing phonetic content that accompanies the facial stimuli. The fusiform gyrus is connected to the lateral anterior temporal gyrus to process information concerning the identity of the person, name and biographical information. These regions would be connected with the amygdala, insula and other structures of the limbic system.

The activation of the amygdala to fearful faces has been extensively demonstrated in neuroimaging studies with healthy volunteers (Breiter et al., 1996) and studies in patients with neurological injuries show that lesions in the amygdala are associated with impairment in the recognition of facial expressions of fear (Adolphs et al., 1994). Although it is quite significant, the relationship between amygdala activation and the expression of fear seems to be unspecific, since it has also been shown activation of this structure to other emotions such as anger (Hariri et al., 2000), disgust (Sprengelmeyer et al., 1998), sadness (Surguladze et al., 2003), happiness (Breiter et al., 1996; Surguladze et al., 2003) and surprise, when this was interpreted negatively (Kim et al., 2003), suggesting a wider role of the amygdala in different stimuli with emotional valence.

The amygdala seems also to be involved in unconscious emotional processes, because neuronal responses has been observed in this area even when the volunteers did not have an explicit recognition of emotional expressions (Whalen et al., 1998). Moreover, the activation of the amygdala to negative facial expressions presented in an unconscious perception paradigm (stimulus presentation for 33 milliseconds, followed by a neutral face, with a duration of 333 milliseconds) was followed by a bias for negative evaluation of the faces in a behavioral paradigm similar to that presented in the scanner (Dannlowski et al., 2007). These findings suggest that the increase in the neuronal activation of the amygdala would correlate with increased identification of emotion.

The processing of facial expressions of disgust has been consistently associated with activations in the insular cortex (Phillips et al., 1997), although negative results and activation of the insula by other emotions such as anger have also been reported. In addition, patients with Huntington's disease has an impairment in the recognition of emotional expressions of disgust (Sprengelmeyer et al., 1996), suggesting that fronto-striatal and especially the basal ganglia are also involved in the recognition of facial expressions of disgust, as these regions are involved in Huntington's disease.

Angry faces can be considered as a guide for the others' behavior, in situations where social rules or expectations are violated (Averill, 1982). The orbitofrontal cortex is crucially involved in this kind of function and activations in this region to expressions of anger are reported (Sprengelmeyer et al., 1998). Additionally, patients with lesions in orbitofrontal cortex, who began to show sociopathic behavior, show a generalized impairment in the recognition of facial expressions, but with a more pronounced impairment in the recognition of faces of anger (Blair, 2003) .

Activations of the frontal cortex and the cingulate cortex during the recognition of various facial expressions can be associated with the function of these regions in cognitive and integrative processing of emotions (Lane et al., 1998).

The processing of facial expressions is predominantly involved in identifying emotions, but there is evidence suggesting that viewing of facial expressions would also be able to evoke emotions through a more primitive emotional contagion (Wild et al., 2001). An alternative to the study of evoked emotions is the use of scenes depicting situations which could lead to subjective emotional states, such as the database developed by Lang and his colleagues (Lang et al., 1993), called the International Affective Picture System (IAPS). Hundreds of scenes constituents of this database were evaluated for the valence and the arousal during the validation process. In a study (Britton et al., 2006) comparing the neuronal activation caused by facial expressions of happiness, sadness, fear and anger with the neuronal activation caused by viewing of IAPS pictures with the same emotional content, it has been shown that both stimuli activated brain areas in common, such as the amygdala, posterior hippocampus, prefrontal cortex and medial visual cortex. Moreover, activations in anterior cingulate, insula and superior temporal gyrus were more pronounced for faces than to scenes. In this study it was found that the agreement on the definition of emotion displayed by the stimulus was greater for faces than for scenes, although the later were rated as with greater valence and arousal than the former. A limitation for the use of scenes would be the complexity and amount of information in each picture, which could lead to the recruitment of additional cognitive processing, and recall of prior personal experiences. On the other hand, habituation would be less frequent with the scenes compared to faces.

The neuroimaging findings indicate the existence of specific neural substrates related to the recognition of facial expressions of basic emotions. A meta-analysis (Phan et al., 2002) suggested that the amygdala plays a key role in processing emotions of fear, while the basal ganglia seem to be particularly involved in processing other emotions such as disgust and happiness. Specifically in regard to the processing of emotional faces, a recent review of 105 fMRI studies with healthy volunteers (Fusar-Poli et al., 2009) has shown activation of amygdala to fearful, happy and sad faces, with a greater sensitivity of the amygdala for fear than happiness or sadness. On the other hand, insular response was observed to angry and disgusted faces, with a greater sensitivity to disgust than to anger. The former meta-analysis also demonstrated that regions of cortex medial prefrontal cortex (areas 9 and 10 of Brodman) extending to the anterior cingulate gyrus (areas 32/33 and 24 of Brodman) are commonly activated by different emotions, strengthening the involvement of these structures in the cognitive aspects of processing of emotions.

Since a considerable body of evidence points to sex differences in the emotional processing (Cahill, 2006), the sexual polymorphism can be a confounding variable in studies looking at the processing of facial expression. Considering the relevance of sex differences in emotional processing, it will be discussed separately.

3. Sexual dimorphism in emotional faces processing

There is a consistent body of evidence of sex differences in the performance of cognitive and emotional functions. In short, women seem to perform better on tasks of verbal fluency, memory and fine motor tasks, while men perform better on tasks related to math and spatial skills (Halpern, 1992). Despite the evidence of sex differences on the cognitive and emotional processes, this issue is still quite controversial and the magnitude, extent and nature of these differences are not fully understood.

Regarding the processing of facial expressions, the results are even more inconsistent. The results of studies comparing the performance of healthy men and women in the identification of basic emotions in facial expressions are controversial, with many pointing to negative results (e.g. Hall et al., 2004), while others point to a difference between the sexes. Among the latter, most of them suggest a better performance of women in the identification of facial expressions, regardless of emotion evaluated (e.g. Hall and Matsumoto, 2004; Rahman et al., 2004; Terracciano et al., 2003). In this direction, physiological parameters suggest a greater responsiveness of women to facial expressions (Campanella et al., 2004; Dimberg, 1990; Orozco & Ehlers, 1998), although negative results have also been reported (Lundqvist, 1995). There are, however, contrary results, showing that men would be faster than women to recognize faces of fear (Campanella et al., 2004) and anger (Williams & Mattingley, 2006).

There is also evidence of sex differences in brain lateralization for the processing of emotions. In general, men use more right hemisphere when processing facial expressions, whereas women use both hemispheres (e.g. Bourne, 2005). Functional neuroimaging studies also suggest a sex difference in the processing of facial expressions (McClure et al., 2004; Williams et al., 2005) and seems to confirm the findings of behavioral lateralization described above. There are, however, reported negative results (Schroeder et al., 2004).

Although neuroimaging studies point to sex differences in neuronal activation caused by emotional faces, results are quite variable, preventing the establishment of a pattern which distinguishes one kind or another. For instance, men showed more pronounced activation of left amygdala in one study (Killgore & Yurgelun-Todd, 2001) but of the right amygdala in other (Williams et al., 2005) to fearful faces. It has also been reported greater activation in right insula and decreased activation in bilateral hippocampus in men during exposure to faces of fear (Williams et al., 2005). Differences in activation of the anterior cingulate cortex are also controversial, with one study showing activation more pronounced in males (McClure et al., 2004) and another study showing higher activation in females (Williams et al., 2005). There is evidence, however, of an interaction between sex of face and sex of the observer in regard to the activations of the anterior cingulate cortex. Men had a more pronounced activation in this region when looking at male faces, whereas women had more pronounced activations viewing female faces (Fischer et al., 2004). Finally, women had greater hemodynamic responses in the amygdala and right frontal regions to the angry faces (McClure et al., 2004) and men showed more pronounced activation of right amygdala to happy faces (Killgore and Yurgelun-Todd, 2001).

Taken together, the behavioral, physiological and neuroimaging data obtained so far indicate a sexual dimorphism in the processing of facial expressions, although the performance data in the paradigms are less consistent.

The difference in the behavioral data may be related to the lack of control of the phase of the menstrual cycle. There is evidence from cognitive studies pointing to a fluctuating response pattern, related to the phases of the menstrual cycle (Maki et al., 2002). In regard to emotional faces, it has also been shown that women identified facial expressions of fear with greater accuracy during the menstrual cycle characterized by high levels of estrogen (Pearson and Lewis, 2005). In addition, higher levels of progesterone have been associated to a better accuracy in the identification of fearful and disgusted faces with averted gaze as more intense than those with direct gaze (Conway et al., 2007). However, conflicting results have also been reported: women in the follicular phase, characterized by lower levels of progesterone, were more accurate in identifying all emotions than women in luteal phase, characterized by higher levels of progesterone. The behavioral performance was associated to stronger amygdalar activation to emotional faces, measured through functional magnetic resonance imaging (fMRI), with a negative correlation between plasma level of progesterone and amygdalar response to fearful, sad and neutral faces (Derntl et al., 2008a; Derntl et al., 2008b). Recently, we have shown that healthy women in the early follicular phase (day 1 to 5 of the menstrual cycle) recognized angry faces more precisely than women in the ovulatory phase (days 12 to 14) or women in the luteal phase (days 21 to 23). Sadness was more accurately recognized by women in the early follicular phase than by women in the luteal phase. Blood levels of estrogen were negatively correlated to the accuracy in identification of angry faces (Guapo et al., 2009).

Overall, the results of the studies carried out so far support the idea that women process facial expressions more efficiently than men. The results of accuracy in the tasks of identifying emotions are supported by physiological measures. For example, women had EEG (Campanella et al., 2004; Orozco and Ehlers, 1998) and EMG (Dimberg, 1990; Lundqvist, 1995) responses more pronounced, reinforcing the hypothesis that women pay more attention and have somatic reactions more intensively to emotional faces. In addition, women take into account the emotion evoked and emotional valence of the stimulus to evaluate facial expressions, while men consider only the valence component (Thayer and Johnsen, 2000). Evidence from the neuroimaging studies suggest that men and women use different neural networks for the processing of emotions, reinforcing the hypothesis of different strategies for the identification of emotions.

Despite the evidence of sex differences in brain function, this variable is rarely controlled in neuroscience research aimed at the cognitive and emotional processes, both normal and pathological (Cahill, 2006). Many mental disorders have a clear sex differences in the prevalence, clinical presentation and response to treatment, making vital controlling this confounding variable in future studies. The prevalence of depression and anxiety disorders is two times higher in women than in men (Kessler et al., 1993; Weissman et al., 1996). However, little attention has been paid to possible sex differences in emotional and cognitive mechanisms involved in the development and maintenance of depressive and anxious symptoms.

4. Anxiety, depression and emotional faces processing

There is evidence that in healthy subjects, some personality traits, which may represent an increased risk for developing depressive or anxiety disorders, may interfere with the processing of facial expressions. The predisposition to react with more anxiety as measured by the trait form of the Trait Anxiety Inventory-State (STAI) (Spielberger, 1983), was associated with a greater accuracy in identifying facial expressions of fear without interfering with the recognition of other facial expressions (Surcinelli et al., 2006). High scores on the Neuroticism subscale of the Personality Questionnaire developed by Hans Eysenck and colleagues have been considered as a vulnerability factor for the occurrence of depression (revised in Christensen & Kessing, 2006. Healthy subjects of both sexes with high scores on the subscale of Neuroticism were less accurate than individuals with low subscale scores in identifying happy faces (Chan et al., 2007).

Physiological measures also confirm changes in processing of faces of fear in anxious individuals (Rossignol et al., 2005). For example, healthy women with high levels of fear of public speaking had a higher sensitivity to angry faces, as measured by contraction of the corrugator muscles, and to happy faces, as measured by contraction of the zygomaticus, and also attributed a more negative valence the faces of anger than women with low fear of public speaking (Dimberg and Thunberg, 2007). Although dysfunctions of the hypothalamic-pituitary-adrenal axis have been reported in patients with depression and anxiety, there is evidence that acutely, glucocorticoids may reduce fear reactions. Acute administration of 40 mg of cortisol attenuated the unconscious perception of facial expressions of fear, particularly in individuals who self-reported themselves as anxious (Putman et al., 2007).

Neuroimaging studies point to a hyperactivity of the amygdala to expressions of fear in individuals with higher levels of anxiety, measured through the scores on the STAI-T (Etkin et al., 2004). Healthy individuals prone to anxiety showed more pronounced activation of the amygdala and insula to faces of anger, fear and happiness compared to a sensorimotor task, than subjects with low propensity to anxiety. No differences were found between the activation caused by each emotion separately (Stein et al., 2007). There is also evidence of an association between the expression of the short allele of the serotonin transporter, which has been associated to a higher risk to depression and anxiety, and hyperreactivity of the amygdala to faces of fear and anger in healthy volunteers of both sexes (Hariri et al., 2002).

Among patients with established diagnosis of anxiety disorders, there is also evidence of impaired processing of facial expressions. Patients with social phobia had higher skin conductance response than healthy volunteers to fearful faces presented subliminally

(Tsunoda et al., 2008). Functional neuroimaging studies have shown that no medicated social phobics patients had more pronounced activation of the amygdala to aversive faces (anger, fear, disgust) compared with faces of happiness, than healthy volunteers, and that the intensity of the hemodynamic response correlated with the severity of the phobic symptoms (Phan et al., 2006).

Panic disorder without agoraphobia or other comorbidities had an impaired of the identification of facial expressions, particularly the emotions of sadness and anger, in comparison to matched healthy controls. Patients also showed a tendency to mistakenly identify other expressions as anger. However, the presence of depressive symptoms correlated with the performance on the task and the difference between patients and controls disappeared when controlled for depression (Kessler et al., 2007). On the other hand, patients diagnosed with panic disorder and homozygous for the 1019G risk allele of the serotonin receptor 5-HT1A type showed more pronounced activation of the amygdala to faces of happiness and attenuation of the activation of prefrontal regions to fearful faces. The same pattern of increased amygdala activation to happy faces was observed in patients carrying the short allele of the serotonin transporter (Domschke et al., 2006).

Compared with healthy controls, panic patients showed lower intensity of the BOLD (Blood Oxygen Level Dependent) signal in the anterior cingulate cortex and amygdala than healthy controls in response to faces of fear and activations of the cingulate cortex were negatively correlated with subjective measures of anxiety (Pillay et al., 2006). This same group demonstrated that in response to faces of happiness, patients with panic disorder showed more pronounced activation of the anterior cingulate cortex, with no differences between groups in amygdalar activations (Pillay et al., 2007).

Some interesting results about emotional processing in patients with anxiety disorder come from a meta-analysis (Etkin & Wager, 2007) aimed at evaluating the functional neuroimaging studies of patients who underwent paradigms characterized by the contrast of negative emotional stimuli with positive or neutral conditions. They included studies with several paradigms and stimuli such as fear of public speaking for social phobia, memory of traumatic events in posttraumatic stress disorder and presentation of phobic stimuli in specific phobia. The processing of facial expressions was assessed in all anxiety disorders. However, panic disorder and obsessive-compulsive disorder were not included in the meta-analysis because the studies conducted so far have not fulfilled the inclusion criteria established by the authors. Activation of the amygdala and insula to negative stimuli were found in the three disorders studied, suggesting a common involvement of these structures in the pathophysiology of these disorders. Hyperactivity of the amygdala and the insula was more frequently observed in social phobia and specific phobia than in posttraumatic stress disorder, which in turn, presented reduced activations in the ventromedial prefrontal cortex, cingulate cortex and thalamus, which was not observed in other mental disorders study.

Cognitive theories tend to imply negative interpretations in the psychopathology of depression. Depressed individuals, or individuals predisposed to depression, have a tendency to evaluate themselves, others and events of everyday life in a more negative way than healthy controls (Beck, 1979). Patients diagnosed with major depression tend to perceive negative emotional stimuli, including faces of sadness, with greater frequency or accuracy than healthy controls, and tend to pay less attention to positive stimuli, such as happy faces. Some of these abnormalities persist after remission of symptoms and are also found in non-depressed persons with a high risk of developing depression (revised in Leppanen, 2006).

Depressed subjects had a negative bias in judging facial expressions (Gur et al., 1992), particularly the emotion of sadness, with a strong correlation with the severity of depressive symptoms (Hale, 1998). In addition, the bias for the judgment of ambiguous facial expressions as sadness seems to be a predictor of the persistence of depressive symptoms (Hale, 1998), particularly in women (Bouhuys et al., 1999). Patients in complete remission from depression had a selective attention to facial expressions of sadness, similar to patients with current depression, while healthy volunteers tend to avoid the sad faces and oriented themselves to faces of happiness (Joormann and Gotlib, 2007). Furthermore, the recognition of facial expressions of fear and higher levels of urinary cortisol in depressed patients in complete remission were predictive of the occurrence of relapse (Bouhuys et al., 2006).

Increased neural activity to negative stimuli and decreased neural activity for positive stimuli in brain regions related to the processing of emotions, such as the amygdala and ventral striatum have also been reported in depressed patients (Leppanen, 2006). Depressed patients showed more pronounced activation of the amygdala and ventral striatum to faces of sadness (Fu et al., 2004) and an attenuated response to faces of happiness in the regions of putamen, hippocampus and ventral striatum compared with healthy controls (Fu et al., 2007). Chronic treatment with antidepressants normalized brain activation, attenuating the neuronal response of the left amygdala and ventral striatum to faces of sadness (Fu et al., 2004) and increasing the response of the ventral striatum to faces of happiness (Fu et al., 2007).

There is also evidence of an association between structural brain changes and emotional faces processing in depressed patients. Individuals diagnosed with major depression showed increased amygdalar volume and reduced hippocampal volume compared to controls, in addition to deficits in learning emotional faces, especially with emotions of fear, surprise and disgust. The size of amygdala correlated with the impairment in task performance and presence of symptoms of anxiety. The size of the hippocampus also correlated with the presence of symptoms of anxiety (Weniger et al., 2006).

Taken together, the studies with patients with depression and anxiety disorders suggest impairment in processing facial expressions of basic emotions. Among anxiety disorders, it has been observed a tendency for greater recognition of negative expressions, especially fear and anger, while in the depressive disorders there is a loss of the recognition of positive expressions and increased recognition of negative expressions, with emphasis in sad faces.

In general, neuroimaging studies indicate greater hemodynamic responses in patients than in healthy controls the presentation of facial expressions of basic emotions. The amygdala has been particularly involved in the pathophysiology of depression and anxiety disorders, and changes in their activation to emotional faces have been found in most studies with psychiatric patients.

5. Pharmacological modulation of emotional faces processing

Other evidence pointing to the existence of distinct neurocognitive systems in the emotional processing come from studies that evaluate the effects of psychoactive drugs in the perception of emotional expressions. Pharmacological challenges that interfere with various neurotransmitter systems have been used for the evaluation of their role in identifying facial expressions, particularly with drugs that act on the serotonergic and GABAergic systems, which will be detailed below.

5.1 Modulation by the serotonergic system

The results of pharmacological challenges that interfere with serotonin function reinforce the role of serotonin (5-HT) in the processing of anxiety and fear (Deakin and Graeff, 1991), and behavioral effects were observed mainly on the recognition of facial expression of fear. Other emotions such as happiness and disgust, also seem to suffer interference in the serotonin levels for processing, though less consistent across studies.

These studies (for review, see Del-Ben et al., 2008) have shown that decreased serotonin function through depletion of the supply of tryptophan in the diet reduced the recognition of facial expressions of fear in women, and in individuals of both sexes carrying the short allele of the serotonin transporter. On the other hand, the acute increase in the dietary intake of tryptophan increased the recognition of expressions of happiness and fear in female volunteers; supplementation of tryptophan for 14 days facilitated the identification of facial expressions of happiness and decreased the recognition of expressions of disgust in women but not in male subjects.

The acute administration of intravenous citalopram, a selective inhibitor of serotonin reuptake inhibitor (SSRI), facilitated the recognition of expressions of happiness and fear in women. A similar effect on faces of fear was obtained after a single dose of citalopram administered orally in healthy volunteers of both sexes. In contrast, the administration for 7 days of oral citalopram (20 mg daily) in healthy volunteers of both sexes has increased the recognition of facial expressions of anger, fear and disgust, compared with the volunteers treated with placebo. A later study from the same group confirmed the reduction of the identification of fearful faces after treatment for 7 days with citalopram (20 mg daily) in both sexes. Euthymic patients with a history of major depression recognized fearful faces more precisely than healthy controls. The acute administration of intravenous citalopram normalized to recognition of expressions of fear in women with a history of depression, but increased the recognition of facial expressions of fear in women with no past history of depression.

These studies also suggest a sexual dimorphism in serotonergic modulation of the perception of facial expressions, since the effects of manipulating serotonin were found mainly in female volunteers. However, it is impossible to explore this hypothesis more deeply, since several studies included only women in their sample.

Acute administration of 3,4-Metilenedioximetamfetamina (MDMA, "ecstasy") in volunteers of both sexes led to an increased recognition of expressions of fear, while in the fourth day of abstinence was observed opposite effect. The drug did not interfere in the recognition of other emotional expressions. Although MDMA causes release of dopamine and norepinephrine, its main mechanism of action is via the serotonergic system, by inhibiting the reuptake of serotonin available in the synaptic cleft and the stimulation of the release of serotonin stored in presynaptic vesicles. In addition, MDMA decreases the synthesis of serotonin by inhibiting the activity of the enzyme tryptophan hydroxylase, leading to a depletion of brain serotonin in the subsequent days of substance use. The acute effect of "ecstasy" facilitated the recognition of facial expressions of fear, but impaired the recognition of facial expressions, four days after use, suggesting that increased 5-HT function facilitates the recognition, while the reduction of 5-HT function enables the perception of facial expressions of fear. Challenges with tryptophan point to the same direction, at least in female subjects. Dietary supplementation of tryptophan, and consequent increased availability of serotonin, facilitated the recognition of facial expressions of fear, while tryptophan depletion impaired the recognition of facial expressions of fear. Acute administration of citalopram facilitated the recognition of facial expressions of fear, an effect similar to those observed with the supplementation of tryptophan in the diet and the acute use of ecstasy and opposite to that observed with the depletion of tryptophan and four days after the use of ecstasy. Taken together, these data suggest an increase in serotonin function immediately after the acute administration of citalopram.

However, in a recent published study (Alves-Neto et al., 2010), we have found a "depressive" effect of a single dose of escitalopram, the pharmacologically active S-enantiomer of RS-citalopram. The R-enantiomer has been shown to reduce the effects of the S-enantiomer (Sanchez, 2006), probably due to negative allosteric interaction at the level of the 5-HT transporter. As result, escitalopram behaves as a highly potent and selective ligand of the 5-HT transporter and clinical studies have shown that escitalopram causes few side effects and has a relatively fast onset of action (Waugh & Goa, 2003). In a placebo controlled crossover design study with healthy male volunteers we have found that a single dose of escitalopram facilitated the recognition of sadness and inhibited the recognition of happiness, but just when viewing male faces.

The interpretation of the effects of acute administration of SSRIs is not simple, since the clinical response to SSRIs is associated with an increase of the serotonin function, which in turn depends on an accommodation of serotonin receptors, particularly a desensitization of presynaptic receptors type 5-HT1A, which occurs after the use of medication for an average of two weeks. It is, therefore, that early treatment with SSRIs would be a reduction of 5-HT function, which can be associated, with the worsening of symptoms commonly seen in patients with anxiety disorders (Kent et al., 1998). Experimental data showed that after acute administration of SSRIs, there is an increase of serotonin in the raphe nuclei that is higher than in cortex (Bel & Artigas, 1992). Therefore, the acute administration of SSRI preferably would increase the concentration of serotonin around the cell bodies of serotonergic neurons, reducing their shots due to the activation of somatodendritics autoreceptors (Gartside et al., 1995), which would lead to a reduction in the post-synaptic serotonin levels. However, microdialysis studies in animals showed increased concentrations of serotonin in the extracellular space in cortical regions after acute administration of SSRI (David et al., 2003). Furthermore, the acute administration of citalopram in healthy volunteers resulted in increased plasma levels of prolactin and cortisol (Attenburrow et al., 2001; McKie et al., 2005), which is considered as an indirect measure of increased levels of serotonin in the central nervous system.

A possible explanation for these apparently contradictory results comes from studies of the functional neuroanatomy of the serotonergic system. These studies have shown that anatomically distinct serotoninergic pathways differently modulate specific brain circuits. These dissociations suggest that serotonin activity within different regions of the raphe nucleus may be under the influence of different regulatory pathways, being recruited in different ways, depending on specific conditions of the environment and the characteristics of the stimulus (Lowry et al., 2005).

5.2 Modulation of the GABAergic system

There is evidence, albeit in smaller numbers, that the GABAergic system also modulates the recognition of basic emotional expressions. Although benzodiazepines are typical anxiolytic drugs, few studies have been carried out so far investigating their effect on the processing of facial expressions, and they show seemingly contradictory results. It has been that 15 mg of diazepam selectively impair the identification of angry faces (Blair & Curran, 1999). In a further study, however, the same research group (Zangara et al., 2002) reported that the same dose of diazepam affected both angry and fearful faces. To explain these conflicting results, the authors considered that the emotional state of the volunteers could have interfered with the processing of emotional cues, since in the former study, the participants reported more anxiety and discomfort than in the latter. Another study has pointed to a global impairment by diazepam of the identification of emotional faces (Coupland et al., 2003). There is also reported evidence showing no effect of lorazepam (Kamboj & Curran, 2006) or of a low dose of diazepam (Murphy et al., 2008) on the recognition of facial emotional expressions.

The discrepancy in results between the studies described above may be due to differences in the interval between drug administration and implementation of the experimental procedure. In the first (Blair & Curran, 1999) and second (Zangara et al., 2002) studies, the task was initiated 40 minutes after ingestion of the drug, while in the third (Coupland et al., 2003), the task began 75 minutes after drug administration. Therefore, the sedative effects of diazepam may have been responsible for a loss of attention and consequent impaired performance on the task. In addition, the sample of the third study (Coupand et al., 2003) was not balanced by sex, with a majority of women relative to men, which may have affected the results, since, as discussed earlier, there is evidence of a sexual dimorphism in processing of emotion.

Although ethanol acts on different neurotransmitter systems, it is known that the GABAergic system is heavily influenced by this substance and therefore the effects of acute alcohol will be discussed in this session. Alcohol impaired the recognition of emotional expressions of anger in women, while men had reduction in the identification of faces of anger, fear and disgust (Borrill et al., 1987). These data reinforce two points raised earlier: a) the GABAergic system plays an important role in the recognition of emotional expressions of anger and b) there is a sexual dimorphism in the recognition of facial expressions. It has also been shown that low doses of alcohol increased, while higher doses of alcohol decreased the recognition of emotional expressions of happiness by healthy males, suggesting a dose-dependent effect of alcohol on the recognition of facial expressions (Kano et al., 2003).

5.3 Pharmacological challenges and functional neuroimaging

The combination of pharmacological challenges with functional magnetic resonance imaging (Pharmacological Functional Magnetic Resonance Imaging, pharmaco fMRI) is an emerging and promising field of study, which allows the investigation of the effect of drugs on cerebral metabolic activity through measures of changes in the BOLD (Blood Oxygen Level Dependent) signal. However, few studies have investigated the modulation of hemodynamic activation by facial expressions.

So far, only one study (Paulus et al., 2005) examined the effects of pharmacological manipulation with benzodiazepines in neuronal activation, measured by magnetic resonance functional, caused by facial expressions of basic emotions. Lorazepam was administered orally, at doses of 0.25 mg and 1 mg in 15 healthy volunteers (six women and nine men). The paradigm of psychological activation consisted of presenting a target face (anger, fear or happiness) at the top of the computer screen, being the volunteers asked to paired the emotional expression of the target face with one of the emotional expressions presented in other two faces shown in bottom the of the computer screen by pressing the right and left of a button box. The control task consisted of matching geometric figures. Regardless of the type of emotion, the volunteers showed activation of bilateral amygdala and insula during the task of matching facial expressions, compared to the control task. Lorazepam attenuated the hemodynamic response of the amygdala and the insula, in a dose-dependent way.

The role of the serotonergic system in the emotional faces processing has been a little more investigated through the association of pharmacological challenges and fMRI.

In an unconscious perception paradigm, where volunteers were asked only to recognize the sex of faces during the imaging acquisition, tryptophan depletion in healthy men increased amygdala activation in response to fear faces compared with neutral and happy faces, but just in individuals with high levels of sensitivity to threat, measured by the BIS/BAS (Behavioral Inhibition System / Behavioral Aversive System) scale (Cools et al., 2005). These results have been replicated in healthy women, showing a significant correlation between sensitivity to threats, as measured by the BIS/BAS scale, and more pronounced activation of the amygdala to fearful faces compared to faces of happiness, under the effect of depletion of tryptophan (van der Veen et al., 2007). This later study also showed that mood changes (depressive symptoms) caused by tryptophan depletion in healthy women with a family history of depression was associated with greater impairment in the performance in a task of sex categorization of faces with negative facial expressions (fear, sadness and disgust) and increased right amygdalar activation to faces of fear.

The effects of tryptophan depletion were also evaluated in the processing of faces of sadness and happiness (Fusar-Poli et al., 2007). Independently of the emotional valence of the face, tryptophan depletion attenuated the activations of the right medial/inferior frontal gyrus, the posterior cingulate cortex, the occipital and parietal cortex bilaterally, the right hippocampus, claustrum and insula. Referring specifically to the amygdala, effects were observed only when the emotions were combined and compared with neutral faces. The depletion of tryptophan attenuated amygdala response to emotional faces.

In a paradigm of sex categorization of faces, we found that a low dose of citalopram (7.5 mg), administered intravenously to healthy male volunteers, attenuated the hemodynamic response in right amygdala and right orbitofrontal cortex to aversive faces (anger, disgust and fear) compared to neutral faces in healthy men (Del-Ben et al., 2005). In a study (Anderson et al., 2007) published latter, we reanalyzed the data evaluating the effects of intravenous citalopram on each emotion separately and found that citalopram attenuated the activation of the amygdala to faces of fear and disgust, while increased activation of the insula to disgust faces. No effects of escitalopram on angry faces have been detected.

In this study (Anderson et al., 2007), although citalopram has reduced the activation of the amygdala to faces of fear and disgust, it occurred in different hemispheres. Possibly this is due to the fact that, regardless of treatment, the right amygdala activation was more robust to the faces of fear, while the left amygdala signal intensity was higher at the faces of disgust. A lateralization of the functions of the amygdala has been suggested; the right amygdala is more associated with arousal and the left with cognitive processes (Skuse et al., 2005). It is possible that the faces of fear have a more immediate emotional salience, while the faces of disgust require the engagement of cognitive functions for their processing. Another possibility would be differences in the time of habituation to the two types of stimuli.

We also observed that, in contrast to the attenuation of the amygdala, citalopram increased the activation of left insula (and on right, at a level below statistical significance), extending to the claustrum, to disgusted faces. The anterior insula has connections with the amygdala and, along with the ventromedial prefrontal cortex, hypothalamus and periaqueductal gray material, is part of a network that modulates the identification and response to threatening stimuli. However, in this study, we found activation of posterior portions of the insula, which seems to be involved with somatosensory processes and pain. Although not specified a priori, citalopram increased the activation of the pulvinar nucleus and occipital cortex, suggesting that serotonin can enhance the function of pathways responsible for the integration of interoceptive and exteroceptive information.

Further studies have confirmed the role of antidepressants in the emotional faces processing. Healthy volunteers of both sexes were subjected to a treatment for seven days with citalopram orally at a dose of 20 mg/day and underwent a paradigm of unconscious perception of facial expressions of fear and happiness marked by the presentation of emotional faces for 17 milliseconds followed by a neutral face with duration of 167 milliseconds. The amygdala was established as a priori region of interest; the treatment caused an attenuation of the activation in the bilateral amygdala to fearful compared with happy faces (Harmer et al., 2006). More recently, the same group has shown that a single dose of citalopram, administered orally, attenuated the amygdalar activation to masked fearful faces (Murphy et al., 2009). Attenuation of amygdala to emotional faces, assessed by a paradigm similar to those used in the lorazepam study (described earlier), has also been obtained with escitalopram, given to health volunteers during 21 days (Arce et al., 2008).

In these neuroimaging studies, effects of the drug in the performance of the tasks performed during the acquisition of neuroimaging were not observed. Also there were no changes in subjective states, except a reduction in self-reported hostility as measured by the Hostility Inventory Buss-Durkee after seven days of use of citalopram.

Given the role of the amygdala in the early stages of coordinating responses to threatening stimuli and the production of emotional states, the effects of citalopram and escitalopram suggest a modulatory role of serotonin in this process, consistent with previous studies showing serotonergic modulation of the amygdala activation to faces of fear by using tryptophan depletion (Cools et al., 2005; van der Veen et al., 2007).

5.4 Combining behavioral data and neuroimaging

To date, few studies have evaluated the modulation of the hemodynamic response caused by facial expressions. In addition, differences in the characteristics of the samples, procedures for acquisition, the analysis of images and paradigms activation employees become even more complex interpreting and conciliating the results of neuroimaging studies.

The interpretation of the modulatory effects of drugs on the findings of fMRI also has its limitations. Increased BOLD signal is considered as an increase rate of neuronal metabolism, as measured by oxygen consumption. The increase in neuronal metabolism caused by the pharmacological challenge may reflect either an increase in performance ("working better") or the need for an extra effort to achieve the same level of function ("working harder"). The ideal experimental design would be studies correlating behavioral and neuroimaging data and taking into account some confounding variables such as dose, route and time of administration of the pharmacological challenges, as well as sex, age, personality traits, previous history of mental disorders of the participant and his/her relatives and genetics.

The only study so far carried out with benzodiazepines (Paulus et al., 2005) pointed to the attenuation of the amygdala and the insula to emotional faces (positive and positive) compared with a sensorimotor task. These data are in line with behavioral data that show an impairment of the recognition of emotional faces, particularly anger, caused by benzodiazepines (Blair and Curran, 1999; Coupland et al., 2003; Zangara et al., 2002).

Conciliating the results obtained in both behavioral studies and neuroimaging findings that evaluated the serotoninergic function makes the situation even more complex, since the direction of the modulation of neuronal activation is contrary to those of the behavioral studies. If indeed there is a direct correlation between neuronal activation and performance on the task, we would expected that increased serotonergic function would increase neuronal activations and vice versa, but the studies carried out so far point to an increase in neuronal activation of the amygdala (Cools et al., 2005; van der Veen et al., 2007) and reduced accuracy in identifying faces of fear (Harmer et al., 2003b; Marsh et al., 2006) under the effect of depletion of tryptophan. Moreover, behavioral studies point to a facilitation, by acute citalopram, of the recognition of faces of fear (Harmer et al., 2003a) and neuroimaging studies show an attenuation of activation of the amygdala with acute dose (Anderson et al., 2007; Murphy et al., 2009) and of citalopram, given during 7 days (Harmer et al., 2006), and escitalopram, given during 21 days (Arce et al., 2008).

The effects of tryptophan depletion described above were obtained only in volunteers sensitive to threat and therefore these apparently contradictory results may be related to the influence of personality traits. As discussed later, clinical studies show a more pronounced activation of the amygdala to facial expressions in healthy subjects with high traits of anxiety and in patients with anxiety disorders.

With regard to citalopram, it may be that the route of administration has some influence on the effects of drugs on serotonin function. As a part of the study described previously (Del-Ben et al., 2005) images were taken immediately before, during and immediately after infusion of citalopram in order to evaluate the direct effects of the drug in the hemodynamic responses. We observed a pattern of activation of neuronal responses in several brain structures involved in emotional processing (McKie et al., 2005) similar to those observed with the administration of metaclorofenilpiperazina (mCPP), a serotonin agonist (Anderson et al., 2002). Therefore, one may speculate that with the intravenous administration, there is an initial effect of increased serotonin function, before the activation of inhibitory auto-receptors. However, the results obtained with a single dose of citalopram, given orally, has also shown an attenuation of amygdala to fearful faces (Murphy et al., 2009).

An alternative explanation for the initial effects of the antidepressants has been proposed by Catherine Harmer and her colleagues (Harmer et al., 2009). It has been proposed that the clinical effects, particularly in depressed patients, are due to initial changes in the way that the individual processes relevant emotional information, correcting the negative emotional bias normally observed in these patients, which, in turn, lead to mood changes. According to this view, early changes in emotional processing precede and contribute to later changes in mood and depressive symptoms following antidepressant drug treatment.

6. Final remarks

Emotional faces processing is an innate and socially relevant human ability that can easily be assessed. It can be under the influence of personality traits, genetics and sexual dimorphism, and can be altered by current or past psychiatric diagnosis. Of particular interest, it can be manipulated by drugs largely used in the clinical practice. Relatively simple paradigms composed by facial expressions of basic emotions have contributed significantly for a better understanding of the pathophysiology of several mental disorders. This tool can also have a role for different purposes, such as the prediction of the clinical response, the discovery of new compounds, among others.

7. References

Adolphs, R., Tranel, D., Damasio, H., Damasio, A., 1994. Impaired recognition of emotion in facial expressions following bilateral damage to the human amygdala. Nature 372, 669-672.

Alves-Neto, W.C., Guapo, V.G., Graeff, F.G., Deakin, J.F., Del-Ben, C.M., 2010. Effect of escitalopram on the processing of emotional faces. Braz J Med Biol Res.

Anderson, I.M., Clark, L., Elliott, R., Kulkarni, B., Williams, S.R., Deakin, J.F., 2002. 5-HT(2C) receptor activation by m-chlorophenylpiperazine detected in humans with fMRI. Neuroreport 13, 1547-1551.

Anderson, I.M., Del-Ben, C.M., McKie, S., Richardson, P., Williams, S.R., Elliott, R., Deakin, J.F., 2007. Citalopram modulation of neuronal responses to aversive face emotions: a functional MRI study. Neuroreport 18, 1351-1355.

Andrew, R.J., 1963. Evolution of Facial Expression. Science 142, 1034-1041.

Arce, E., Simmons, A.N., Lovero, K.L., Stein, M.B., Paulus, M.P., 2008. Escitalopram effects on insula and amygdala BOLD activation during emotional processing. Psychopharmacology (Berl) 196, 661-672.

Attenburrow, M.J., Mitter, P.R., Whale, R., Terao, T., Cowen, P.J., 2001. Low-dose citalopram as a 5-HT neuroendocrine probe. Psychopharmacology (Berl) 155, 323-326.

Averill, J.R., 1982. Anger and aggression: an essay of emotion, New York.

Beck, A.T., 1979. Cognitive therapy of depression. Guilford Press, New York.

Bel, N., Artigas, F., 1992. Fluvoxamine preferentially increases extracellular 5-hydroxytryptamine in the raphe nuclei: an in vivo microdialysis study. Eur J Pharmacol 229, 101-103.

Blair, R.J., 2003. Neurobiological basis of psychopathy. Br J Psychiatry 182, 5-7.

Blair, R.J., Curran, H.V., 1999. Selective impairment in the recognition of anger induced by diazepam. Psychopharmacology (Berl) 147, 335-338.

Borrill, J.A., Rosen, B.K., Summerfield, A.B., 1987. The influence of alcohol on judgement of facial expression of emotion. Br J Med Psychol 60 (Pt 1), 71-77.

Bouhuys, A.L., Bos, E.H., Geerts, E., van Os, T.W., Ormel, J., 2006. The association between levels of cortisol secretion and fear perception in patients with remitted depression predicts recurrence. J Nerv Ment Dis 194, 478-484.

Bouhuys, A.L., Geerts, E., Gordijn, M.C., 1999. Depressed patients' perceptions of facial emotions in depressed and remitted states are associated with relapse: a longitudinal study. J Nerv Ment Dis 187, 595-602.

Bourne, V.J., 2005. Lateralised processing of positive facial emotion: sex differences in strength of hemispheric dominance. Neuropsychologia 43, 953-956.

Breiter, H.C., Etcoff, N.L., Whalen, P.J., Kennedy, W.A., Rauch, S.L., Buckner, R.L., Strauss, M.M., Hyman, S.E., Rosen, B.R., 1996. Response and habituation of the human amygdala during visual processing of facial expression. Neuron 17, 875-887.

Britton, J.C., Taylor, S.F., Sudheimer, K.D., Liberzon, I., 2006. Facial expressions and complex IAPS pictures: common and differential networks. Neuroimage 31, 906-919.

Cahill, L., 2006. Why sex matters for neuroscience. Nat Rev Neurosci 7, 477-484.

Campanella, S., Rossignol, M., Mejias, S., Joassin, F., Maurage, P., Debatisse, D., Bruyer, R., Crommelinck, M., Guerit, J.M., 2004. Human gender differences in an emotional visual oddball task: an event-related potentials study. Neurosci Lett 367, 14-18.

Chan, S.W., Goodwin, G.M., Harmer, C.J., 2007. Highly neurotic never-depressed students have negative biases in information processing. Psychol Med 37, 1281-1291.

Christensen, M.V., Kessing, L.V., 2006. Do personality traits predict first onset in depressive and bipolar disorder? Nord J Psychiatry 60, 79-88.

Conway, C.A., Jones, B.C., DeBruine, L.M., Welling, L.L., Law Smith, M.J., Perrett, D.I., Sharp, M.A., Al-Dujaili, E.A., 2007. Salience of emotional displays of danger and contagion in faces is enhanced when progesterone levels are raised. Horm Behav 51, 202-206.

Cools, R., Calder, A.J., Lawrence, A.D., Clark, L., Bullmore, E., Robbins, T.W., 2005. Individual differences in threat sensitivity predict serotonergic modulation of amygdala response to fearful faces. Psychopharmacology (Berl) 180, 670-679.

Coupland, N.J., Singh, A.J., Sustrik, R.A., Ting, P., Blair, R., 2003. Effects of diazepam on facial emotion recognition. J Psychiatry Neurosci 28, 452-463.

Dannlowski, U., Ohrmann, P., Bauer, J., Kugel, H., Arolt, V., Heindel, W., Suslow, T., 2007. Amygdala reactivity predicts automatic negative evaluations for facial emotions. Psychiatry Res 154, 13-20.

Darwin, C., 1872. The expression of the emotions in man and animals. Murray, [S.l.].

David, D.J., Bourin, M., Jego, G., Przybylski, C., Jolliet, P., Gardier, A.M., 2003. Effects of acute treatment with paroxetine, citalopram and venlafaxine in vivo on noradrenaline and serotonin outflow: a microdialysis study in Swiss mice. Br J Pharmacol 140, 1128-1136.

Deakin, J.F.W., Graeff, F.G., 1991. 5-HT and mechanisms of defense. Journal of Psychopharmacology 5, 10.

Del-Ben, C.M., Deakin, J.F., McKie, S., Delvai, N.A., Williams, S.R., Elliott, R., Dolan, M., Anderson, I.M., 2005. The effect of citalopram pretreatment on neuronal responses to neuropsychological tasks in normal volunteers: an FMRI study. Neuropsychopharmacology 30, 1724-1734.

Del-Ben, C.M., Ferreira, C.A., Alves-Neto, W.C., Graeff, F.G., 2008. Serotonergic modulation of face-emotion recognition. Braz J Med Biol Res 41, 263-269.

Derntl, B., Kryspin-Exner, I., Fernbach, E., Moser, E., Habel, U., 2008a. Emotion recognition accuracy in healthy young females is associated with cycle phase. Horm Behav 53, 90-95.

Derntl, B., Windischberger, C., Robinson, S., Lamplmayr, E., Kryspin-Exner, I., Gur, R.C., Moser, E., Habel, U., 2008b. Facial emotion recognition and amygdala activation are associated with menstrual cycle phase. Psychoneuroendocrinology 33, 1031-1040.

Dimberg, U., 1990. Facial electromyography and emotional reactions. Psychophysiology 27, 481-494.

Dimberg, U., Thunberg, M., 2007. Speech anxiety and rapid emotional reactions to angry and happy facial expressions. Scand J Psychol 48, 321-328.

Domschke, K., Braun, M., Ohrmann, P., Suslow, T., Kugel, H., Bauer, J., Hohoff, C., Kersting, A., Engelien, A., Arolt, V., Heindel, W., Deckert, J., 2006. Association of the functional -1019C/G 5-HT1A polymorphism with prefrontal cortex and amygdala activation measured with 3 T fMRI in panic disorder. Int J Neuropsychopharmacol 9, 349-355.

Ekman, P., Friesen, F., 1976. Pictures of Facial Affect. Consulting Psychology, Palo Alto, California.

Ekman, P., Sorenson, E.R., Friesen, W.V., 1969. Pan-cultural elements in facial displays of emotion. Science 164, 86-88.

Etkin, A., Klemenhagen, K.C., Dudman, J.T., Rogan, M.T., Hen, R., Kandel, E.R., Hirsch, J., 2004. Individual differences in trait anxiety predict the response of the basolateral amygdala to unconsciously processed fearful faces. Neuron 44, 1043-1055.

Etkin, A., Wager, T.D., 2007. Functional neuroimaging of anxiety: a meta-analysis of emotional processing in PTSD, social anxiety disorder, and specific phobia. Am J Psychiatry 164, 1476-1488.

Fischer, H., Fransson, P., Wright, C.I., Backman, L., 2004. Enhanced occipital and anterior cingulate activation in men but not in women during exposure to angry and fearful male faces. Cogn Affect Behav Neurosci 4, 326-334.

Fu, C.H., Williams, S.C., Brammer, M.J., Suckling, J., Kim, J., Cleare, A.J., Walsh, N.D., Mitterschiffthaler, M.T., Andrew, C.M., Pich, E.M., Bullmore, E.T., 2007. Neural responses to happy facial expressions in major depression following antidepressant treatment. Am J Psychiatry 164, 599-607.

Fu, C.H., Williams, S.C., Cleare, A.J., Brammer, M.J., Walsh, N.D., Kim, J., Andrew, C.M., Pich, E.M., Williams, P.M., Reed, L.J., Mitterschiffthaler, M.T., Suckling, J., Bullmore, E.T., 2004. Attenuation of the neural response to sad faces in major depression by antidepressant treatment: a prospective, event-related functional magnetic resonance imaging study. Arch Gen Psychiatry 61, 877-889.

Fusar-Poli, P., Placentino, A., Carletti, F., Landi, P., Allen, P., Surguladze, S., Benedetti, F., Abbamonte, M., Gasparotti, R., Barale, F., Perez, J., McGuire, P., Politi, P., 2009. Functional atlas of emotional faces processing: a voxel-based meta-analysis of 105 functional magnetic resonance imaging studies. J Psychiatry Neurosci 34, 418-432.

Gartside, S.E., Umbers, V., Hajos, M., Sharp, T., 1995. Interaction between a selective 5-HT1A receptor antagonist and an SSRI in vivo: effects on 5-HT cell firing and extracellular 5-HT. Br J Pharmacol 115, 1064-1070.

Guapo, V.G., Graeff, F.G., Zani, A.C., Labate, C.M., dos Reis, R.M., Del-Ben, C.M., 2009. Effects of sex hormonal levels and phases of the menstrual cycle in the processing of emotional faces. Psychoneuroendocrinology 34, 1087-1094.

Gur, R.C., Erwin, R.J., Gur, R.E., Zwil, A.S., Heimberg, C., Kraemer, H.C., 1992. Facial emotion discrimination: II. Behavioral findings in depression. Psychiatry Res 42, 241-251.

Gur, R.C., Sara, R., Hagendoorn, M., Marom, O., Hughett, P., Macy, L., Turner, T., Bajcsy, R., Posner, A., Gur, R.E., 2002. A method for obtaining 3-dimensional facial expressions and its standardization for use in neurocognitive studies. J Neurosci Methods 115, 137-143.

Hale, W.W., 3rd, 1998. Judgment of facial expressions and depression persistence. Psychiatry Res 80, 265-274.

Hall, C.W., Gaul, L., Kent, M., 1999. College students' perception of facial expressions. Percept Mot Skills 89, 763-770.

Hall, J.A., Matsumoto, D., 2004. Gender differences in judgments of multiple emotions from facial expressions. Emotion 4, 201-206.

Halpern, D.F., 1992. Sex differences in cognitive abilities, 2nd ed, Hillsdale, NJ.

Hariri, A.R., Bookheimer, S.Y., Mazziotta, J.C., 2000. Modulating emotional responses: effects of a neocortical network on the limbic system. Neuroreport 11, 43-48.

Hariri, A.R., Mattay, V.S., Tessitore, A., Kolachana, B., Fera, F., Goldman, D., Egan, M.F., Weinberger, D.R., 2002. Serotonin transporter genetic variation and the response of the human amygdala. Science 297, 400-403.

Harmer, C.J., Bhagwagar, Z., Perrett, D.I., Vollm, B.A., Cowen, P.J., Goodwin, G.M., 2003a. Acute SSRI administration affects the processing of social cues in healthy volunteers. Neuropsychopharmacology 28, 148-152.

Harmer, C.J., Goodwin, G.M., Cowen, P.J., 2009. Why do antidepressants take so long to work? A cognitive neuropsychological model of antidepressant drug action. Br J Psychiatry 195, 102-108.

Harmer, C.J., Mackay, C.E., Reid, C.B., Cowen, P.J., Goodwin, G.M., 2006. Antidepressant drug treatment modifies the neural processing of nonconscious threat cues. Biol Psychiatry 59, 816-820.

Harmer, C.J., Rogers, R.D., Tunbridge, E., Cowen, P.J., Goodwin, G.M., 2003b. Tryptophan depletion decreases the recognition of fear in female volunteers. Psychopharmacology (Berl) 167, 411-417.

Haxby, J.V., Hoffman, E.A., Gobbini, M.I., 2002. Human neural systems for face recognition and social communication. Biol Psychiatry 51, 59-67.

Joormann, J., Gotlib, I.H., 2007. Selective attention to emotional faces following recovery from depression. J Abnorm Psychol 116, 80-85.

Kamboj, S.K., Curran, H.V., 2006. Scopolamine induces impairments in the recognition of human facial expressions of anger and disgust. Psychopharmacology (Berl) 185, 529-535.

Kano, M., Gyoba, J., Kamachi, M., Mochizuki, H., Hongo, M., Yanai, K., 2003. Low doses of alcohol have a selective effect on the recognition of happy facial expressions. Hum Psychopharmacol 18, 131-139.

Kent, J.M., Coplan, J.D., Gorman, J.M., 1998. Clinical utility of the selective serotonin reuptake inhibitors in the spectrum of anxiety. Biol Psychiatry 44, 812-824.

Kesler-West, M.L., Andersen, A.H., Smith, C.D., Avison, M.J., Davis, C.E., Kryscio, R.J., Blonder, L.X., 2001. Neural substrates of facial emotion processing using fMRI. Brain Res Cogn Brain Res 11, 213-226.

Kessler, H., Roth, J., von Wietersheim, J., Deighton, R.M., Traue, H.C., 2007. Emotion recognition patterns in patients with panic disorder. Depress Anxiety 24, 223-226.

Kessler, R.C., McGonagle, K.A., Swartz, M., Blazer, D.G., Nelson, C.B., 1993. Sex and depression in the National Comorbidity Survey. I: Lifetime prevalence, chronicity and recurrence. J Affect Disord 29, 85-96.

Killgore, W.D., Yurgelun-Todd, D.A., 2001. Sex differences in amygdala activation during the perception of facial affect. Neuroreport 12, 2543-2547.

Kim, H., Somerville, L.H., Johnstone, T., Alexander, A.L., Whalen, P.J., 2003. Inverse amygdala and medial prefrontal cortex responses to surprised faces. Neuroreport 14, 2317-2322.

Lane, R.D., Reiman, E.M., Axelrod, B., Yun, L.S., Holmes, A., Schwartz, G.E., 1998. Neural correlates of levels of emotional awareness. Evidence of an interaction between emotion and attention in the anterior cingulate cortex. J Cogn Neurosci 10, 525-535.

Lang, P.J., Greenwald, M.K., Bradley, M.M., Hamm, A.O., 1993. Looking at pictures: affective, facial, visceral, and behavioral reactions. Psychophysiology 30, 261-273.

Leppanen, J.M., 2006. Emotional information processing in mood disorders: a review of behavioral and neuroimaging findings. Curr Opin Psychiatry 19, 34-39.

Lowry, C.A., Johnson, P.L., Hay-Schmidt, A., Mikkelsen, J., Shekhar, A., 2005. Modulation of anxiety circuits by serotonergic systems. Stress 8, 233-246.

Lundqvist, L.O., 1995. Facial EMG reactions to facial expressions: a case of facial emotional contagion? Scand J Psychol 36, 130-141.

Maki, P.M., Rich, J.B., Rosenbaum, R.S., 2002. Implicit memory varies across the menstrual cycle: estrogen effects in young women. Neuropsychologia 40, 518-529.

Marsh, A.A., Finger, E.C., Buzas, B., Soliman, N., Richell, R.A., Vythilingham, M., Pine, D.S., Goldman, D., Blair, R.J., 2006. Impaired recognition of fear facial expressions in 5-HTTLPR S-polymorphism carriers following tryptophan depletion. Psychopharmacology (Berl) 189, 387-394.

McClure, E.B., Monk, C.S., Nelson, E.E., Zarahn, E., Leibenluft, E., Bilder, R.M., Charney, D.S., Ernst, M., Pine, D.S., 2004. A developmental examination of gender differences in brain engagement during evaluation of threat. Biol Psychiatry 55, 1047-1055.

McKie, S., Del-Ben, C., Elliott, R., Williams, S., del Vai, N., Anderson, I., Deakin, J.F., 2005. Neuronal effects of acute citalopram detected by pharmacoMRI. Psychopharmacology (Berl) 180, 680-686.

Murphy, S.E., Downham, C., Cowen, P.J., Harmer, C.J., 2008. Direct effects of diazepam on emotional processing in healthy volunteers. Psychopharmacology (Berl) 199, 503-513.

Murphy, S.E., Norbury, R., O'Sullivan, U., Cowen, P.J., Harmer, C.J., 2009. Effect of a single dose of citalopram on amygdala response to emotional faces. Br J Psychiatry 194, 535-540.

Öhman, A., 2002. Automaticity and the Amygdala: Nonconscious Responses to Emotional Faces. Current Directions in Psychological Sciences, p. 5.

Orozco, S., Ehlers, C.L., 1998. Gender differences in electrophysiological responses to facial stimuli. Biol Psychiatry 44, 281-289.

Paulus, M.P., Feinstein, J.S., Castillo, G., Simmons, A.N., Stein, M.B., 2005. Dose-dependent decrease of activation in bilateral amygdala and insula by lorazepam during emotion processing. Arch Gen Psychiatry 62, 282-288.

Pearson, R., Lewis, M.B., 2005. Fear recognition across the menstrual cycle. Horm Behav 47, 267-271.

Phan, K.L., Fitzgerald, D.A., Nathan, P.J., Tancer, M.E., 2006. Association between amygdala hyperactivity to harsh faces and severity of social anxiety in generalized social phobia. Biol Psychiatry 59, 424-429.

Phan, K.L., Wager, T., Taylor, S.F., Liberzon, I., 2002. Functional neuroanatomy of emotion: a meta-analysis of emotion activation studies in PET and fMRI. Neuroimage 16, 331-348.

Phillips, M.L., Young, A.W., Senior, C., Brammer, M., Andrew, C., Calder, A.J., Bullmore, E.T., Perrett, D.I., Rowland, D., Williams, S.C., Gray, J.A., David, A.S., 1997. A specific neural substrate for perceiving facial expressions of disgust. Nature 389, 495-498.

Pillay, S.S., Gruber, S.A., Rogowska, J., Simpson, N., Yurgelun-Todd, D.A., 2006. fMRI of fearful facial affect recognition in panic disorder: the cingulate gyrus-amygdala connection. J Affect Disord 94, 173-181.

Pillay, S.S., Rogowska, J., Gruber, S.A., Simpson, N., Yurgelun-Todd, D.A., 2007. Recognition of happy facial affect in panic disorder: an fMRI study. J Anxiety Disord 21, 381-393.

Putman, P., Hermans, E.J., Koppeschaar, H., van Schijndel, A., van Honk, J., 2007. A single administration of cortisol acutely reduces preconscious attention for fear in anxious young men. Psychoneuroendocrinology 32, 793-802.

Rahman, Q., Wilson, G.D., Abrahams, S., 2004. Sex, sexual orientation, and identification of positive and negative facial affect. Brain Cogn 54, 179-185.

Rossignol, M., Philippot, P., Douilliez, C., Crommelinck, M., Campanella, S., 2005. The perception of fearful and happy facial expression is modulated by anxiety: an event-related potential study. Neurosci Lett 377, 115-120.

Russell, J.A., 1994. Is there universal recognition of emotion from facial expression? A review of the cross-cultural studies. Psychol Bull 115, 102-141.

Sanchez, C., 2006. The pharmacology of citalopram enantiomers: the antagonism by R-citalopram on the effect of S-citalopram. Basic Clin Pharmacol Toxicol 99, 91-95.

Schroeder, U., Hennenlotter, A., Erhard, P., Haslinger, B., Stahl, R., Lange, K.W., Ceballos-Baumann, A.O., 2004. Functional neuroanatomy of perceiving surprised faces. Hum Brain Mapp 23, 181-187.

Skuse, D.H., Morris, J.S., Dolan, R.J., 2005. Functional dissociation of amygdala-modulated arousal and cognitive appraisal, in Turner syndrome. Brain 128, 2084-2096.

Spielberger, C.D., 1983. Manual for the state/trait anxiety inventory (form Y) : (self evaluation questionnaire). Consulting Psychologists Press, Palo Alto.

Sprengelmeyer, R., Rausch, M., Eysel, U.T., Przuntek, H., 1998. Neural structures associated with recognition of facial expressions of basic emotions. Proc Biol Sci 265, 1927-1931.

Sprengelmeyer, R., Young, A.W., Calder, A.J., Karnat, A., Lange, H., Homberg, V., Perrett, D.I., Rowland, D., 1996. Loss of disgust. Perception of faces and emotions in Huntington's disease. Brain 119 (Pt 5), 1647-1665.

Stein, M.B., Simmons, A.N., Feinstein, J.S., Paulus, M.P., 2007. Increased amygdala and insula activation during emotion processing in anxiety-prone subjects. Am J Psychiatry 164, 318-327.

Surcinelli, P., Codispoti, M., Montebarocci, O., Rossi, N., Baldaro, B., 2006. Facial emotion recognition in trait anxiety. J Anxiety Disord 20, 110-117.

Surguladze, S.A., Brammer, M.J., Young, A.W., Andrew, C., Travis, M.J., Williams, S.C., Phillips, M.L., 2003. A preferential increase in the extrastriate response to signals of danger. Neuroimage 19, 1317-1328.

Terracciano, A., Merritt, M., Zonderman, A.B., Evans, M.K., 2003. Personality traits and sex differences in emotion recognition among African Americans and Caucasians. Ann N Y Acad Sci 1000, 309-312.

Thayer, J.F., Johnsen, B.H., 2000. Sex differences in judgement of facial affect: a multivariate analysis of recognition errors. Scand J Psychol 41, 243-246.

Tsunoda, T., Yoshino, A., Furusawa, T., Miyazaki, M., Takahashi, Y., Nomura, S., 2008. Social anxiety predicts unconsciously provoked emotional responses to facial expression. Physiol Behav 93, 172-176.

van der Veen, F.M., Evers, E.A., Deutz, N.E., Schmitt, J.A., 2007. Effects of acute tryptophan depletion on mood and facial emotion perception related brain activation and performance in healthy women with and without a family history of depression. Neuropsychopharmacology 32, 216-224.

Waugh, J., Goa, K.L., 2003. Escitalopram : a review of its use in the management of major depressive and anxiety disorders. CNS Drugs 17, 343-362.

Weissman, M.M., Bland, R.C., Canino, G.J., Faravelli, C., Greenwald, S., Hwu, H.G., Joyce, P.R., Karam, E.G., Lee, C.K., Lellouch, J., Lepine, J.P., Newman, S.C., Rubio-Stipec, M., Wells, J.E., Wickramaratne, P.J., Wittchen, H., Yeh, E.K., 1996. Cross-national epidemiology of major depression and bipolar disorder. JAMA 276, 293-299.

Weniger, G., Lange, C., Irle, E., 2006. Abnormal size of the amygdala predicts impaired emotional memory in major depressive disorder. J Affect Disord 94, 219-229.

Whalen, P.J., Rauch, S.L., Etcoff, N.L., McInerney, S.C., Lee, M.B., Jenike, M.A., 1998. Masked presentations of emotional facial expressions modulate amygdala activity without explicit knowledge. J Neurosci 18, 411-418.

Wild, B., Erb, M., Bartels, M., 2001. Are emotions contagious? Evoked emotions while viewing emotionally expressive faces: quality, quantity, time course and gender differences. Psychiatry Res 102, 109-124.

Williams, L.M., Barton, M.J., Kemp, A.H., Liddell, B.J., Peduto, A., Gordon, E., Bryant, R.A., 2005. Distinct amygdala-autonomic arousal profiles in response to fear signals in healthy males and females. Neuroimage 28, 618-626.

Williams, M.A., Mattingley, J.B., 2006. Do angry men get noticed? Curr Biol 16, R402-404.

Zangara, A., Blair, R.J., Curran, H.V., 2002. A comparison of the effects of a beta-adrenergic blocker and a benzodiazepine upon the recognition of human facial expressions. Psychopharmacology (Berl) 163, 36-41.

4

Challenges for PET Neuroimaging of Depressive Disorders

Donald F. Smith[a,c] and Philip W. Miller[b,c]

[a] *Center for Psychiatric Research, Psychiatric Hospital of Aarhus University, 8240 Risskov, Denmark*

[b] *Department of Chemistry, Imperial College London, South Kensington, London, SW7 2AZ, England*

[c] *PET Center, Aarhus University Hospital, 8000 C Aarhus, Denmark*

1. Introduction

This chapter deals with two major challenges facing PET neuroimaging of depressive disorders: determining the neurobiology of depressive disorders and inventing suitable positron-emitting radioligands for exploring molecular aspects of brain function. Over the years, PET neuroimaging of depressive disorder has focused almost exclusively on monoaminergic neurotransmission, but judging from recent reports, those studies have failed to demonstrate reliable links between either serotonergic or dopaminergic mechanisms and depressive disorders. Today, disturbances in numerous other neurobiological processes are thought to cause depressive disorder, but we lack PET radioligands to test most modern hypotheses in the living human brain. Thus, the future success of PET neuroimaging of depressive disorders depends on advances in neuroscience concerning molecular neurobiology and on advances in radiochemistry for the synthesis of novel positron-emitting molecules to test hypotheses on the neurobiology of depressive disorders. Success in PET neuroimaging of depressive disorders is expected to provide insight toward better prevention and treatment of these disabling conditions.

2. Depressive disorders

Depression is a severe, disabling, and sometime fatal illness. Symptoms of depression include a mental state of hopelessness, sleep disturbance, altered appetite, lack of energy, concentration difficulties, low self-esteem, self-destructive behavior, painful bodily sensations, and suicidal ideation. Needless to say, depressive disorders require prompt attention and appropriate care. A major current issue in psychiatry is the lack effective treatments to relieve the symptoms of depression in many sufferers (Berlim et al. 2008;Rush et al. 2003a;Rush et al. 2009). Hopefully, further studies of neurobiological mechanisms in depressive disorders will eventually lead to more effective antidepressant treatments. That hope has motivated many studies of molecular mechanisms in depression using positron emission tomography (PET).

3. Principles of PET neuroimaging

PET neuroimaging is a challenging technology. It requires rapid synthesis of highly-purified positron-emitting radioligands of high specific activity, intravenous injection of radioactive compound often with arterial blood sampling in partially immobilized subjects, 3-dimensional registration of photon emissions from the target organ over time, and computerized computations of kinetic parameters. The kinetic parameter used most often to describe the outcome of PET neuroimaging, namely the binding potential, is a complex entity composed of three factors: the number of receptors that are available for binding by the PET radioligand, the affinity of the available receptors toward the PET radioligand , and the concentration of molecules other than the PET radioligand that bind to those receptors (Dunlop and Nemeroff 2007;Laruelle 2000;Lammertsma 2002). The binding potential is an estimate that reflects a series of molecular events, and its value depends on the kinetic model selected for the data analysis. The contribution of individual factors to the binding potential cannot be determined by the single-scan design used in most PET studies of depression. Thus, the complexity of both depression and PET sets limits on the interpretation of findings.

Most PET studies of depressive disorders have been based on the monoamine hypothesis (Schildkraut et al. 1968;Schildkraut and Kety 1967), despite the clear-cut need for exploring other strategies (Hindmarch 2002;Berton and Nestler 2006;Pittenger and Duman 2008;Paschos et al. 2009;Covington, III et al. 2010;Wegener and Volke 2010). Here, we first review recent molecular PET reports on depressive disorders in humans. Next, we discuss challenges for PET in studying in humans the molecular basis of depressive disorders. Then, we outline the need for suitable positron-emitting radioligands for testing modern hypotheses on the causes and consequences of depressive disorders. Clearly, there are a number of major challenges facing those who care to know the molecular basis of these disabling and sometimes fatal diseases.

4. Recent PET studies of serotonin in depressive disorders

Serotonergic neurotransmission has received most attention in studies of depression (Nemeroff and Owens 2009;Owens and Nemeroff 1994). We find, however, that PET studies have not provided consistent findings of a causal link between serotonergic dysfunction and the severity of depressive disorders. Ten PET studies published in recent years have used [^{11}C]McNeil 5652 or [^{11}C]DASB to assess the serotonin transporter in depressed subjects and healthy controls. Four of those studies, plus a data re-analysis, noted less binding by the serotonin transporter in brain regions of depressed subjects (Miller et al. 2008;Oquendo et al. 2007;Parsey et al. 2006a;Reimold et al. 2008;Miller et al. 2009b), four studies found more binding by the serotonin transporter in depressed subjects (Reivich et al. 2004;Cannon et al. 2006b;Cannon et al. 2007;Boileau et al. 2008), and two studies found no difference between depressed subjects and healthy controls in binding by serotonin transporters in brain regions (Meyer et al. 2004;Bhagwagar et al. 2007).

Discrepancies are also apparent in the outcome of recent PET studies carried out with [^{11}C]WAY-100635 or [^{18}F]FCWAY to assess serotonin type 1A receptors in depressed subjects and healthy controls. Here, five studies noted less binding by serotonin type 1A receptors in brain regions of depressed subjects (Bhagwagar et al. 2004;Meltzer et al. 2004;Hirvonen et al. 2008;Drevets et al. 2007;Theodore et al. 2007), one study reported no difference between depressed subjects and healthy controls in binding by serotonin type 1A receptors (Mickey et al. 2008), while more binding by serotonin type 1A receptors was found in three studies of depressed subjects or remitted, depressed subjects compared with healthy controls, with no correlation between receptor binding and depression severity (Parsey et al. 2006b;Miller et al. 2009a;Sullivan et al. 2009). In addition, neither antidepressant treatment including ECT nor induction of depression by depletion of tryptophan affected binding by serotonin type 1A receptors in brain regions (Moses-Kolko et al. 2007;Praschak-Rieder et al. 2004;Saijo et al. 2010). These findings clearly challenge the notion that alterations of serotonergic functions are causally linked with either depressive disorders or antidepressant efficacy.

Serotonin type 2 receptors have also been studied by PET in recent years in relation to depressive disorders. Two closely-related studies used [^{18}F]altanserin for PET and noted less hippocampal binding in depressed subjects than in healthy controls (Mintun et al. 2004;Sheline et al. 2004). In contrast, two other PET studies used either [^{11}C]MDL 100,907 or [^{18}F]setoperone to assess serotonin type 2 receptors and noted more binding in depressive subjects than in healthy controls (Bhagwagar et al. 2006;Meyer et al. 2003). In our view, PET studies with the radioligands that are currently available for assessing serotonergic functions in the living human brain have failed to provide conclusive evidence for aberrant serotonergic mechanisms in depressive disorders. We have noted, however, that receptor occupancy of serotonin transporters can be assessed reliably by PET with [^{11}C]DASB or [^{11}C]McNeil 5652 (Voineskos et al. 2007;Miller et al. 2008). Perhaps studies of receptor occupancy before and during antidepressant therapies can provide a means of determining whether treatment-resistance stems from inadequate receptor blockade.

Monoamine oxidase has also received attention in PET studies of depressive disorders. One study used [^{11}C]harmine, a reversible inhibitor of type A MAO, for PET scanning in order to see whether the activity of that enzyme differs between depressed patients and healthy subjects (Meyer et al. 2006a). More binding of [^{11}C]harmine was noted in brain regions of depressed patients than in healthy controls, but no correlation was found between clinical variables and PET findings in the patients. A lack of correspondence between clinical condition of patients and degree of binding of [^{11}C]harmine in brain regions was also observed in a recent follow-up PET study of type A MAO in depressive disorders; an elevated distribution volume of the PET radioligand persisted in patients despite symptom-reduction during antidepressant drug treatment (Meyer et al. 2009a).

5. Recent PET studies of dopamine in depressive disorders

Dopaminergic neurotransmission is thought to play a role in depression, perhaps via defects in central reward systems (Randrup and Braestrup 1977;Spanagel and Weiss 1999). Several PET radioligands have been used in recent years for probing dopaminergic mechanisms in depressed humans. [^{18}F]Fluoro-L-dopa is used routinely for assessing dopamine synthesis by PET in Parkinson's disease (Takikawa et al. 1994), and it showed reduced striatal uptake in depressed subjects with retarded movement (Bragulat et al. 2007). Certain dopamine receptors have also been examined by PET in recent years in depressed subjects. Dopamine D_1 receptors were assessed by [^{11}C]SCH 23,390 or [^{11}C]NNC-112 in two PET studies of depression (Dougherty et al. 2006;Cannon et al. 2008), and both reports found less binding in striatal regions of depressed subjects than of healthy controls. Dopamine $D_{2/3}$ receptors have been assessed in five PET studies using either [^{11}C]raclopride or [^{11}C]FLB 457 in depressed subjects and healthy controls; one study noted more striatal binding by dopamine $D_{2/3}$ receptors in depressed subjects (Meyer et al. 2006b), another study found less dopamine $D_{2/3}$ receptor binding in depression (Montgomery et al. 2007), and three studies showed no difference between depressed and healthy subjects in dopamine $D_{2/3}$ receptor binding in brain regions (Kuroda et al. 2006;Montgomery et al. 2007;Busto et al. 2009). The transport of dopamine as well as noradrenaline from the synaptic cleft into presynaptic terminals was assessed by PET using [^{11}C]RTI-32 in 20 Parkinson patients, some of which were depressed (Remy et al. 2005). Less transporter binding was noted in brain regions of depressed Parkinson patients than of non-depressed patients with Parkinson's disease. In our view, a consistent picture of causal relationships between dopaminergic disturbances and depression has failed to appear from PET studies carried out with the positron-emitting radioligands that are currently available for use in humans, except perhaps for movement disorders of depressed subjects.

6. Recent PET neuroimaging of non-serotonergic and non-dopaminergic mechanisms in depressive disorders.

Relatively few PET studies of depressive disorders have been reported recently on molecular mechanisms unrelated to serotonergic and dopaminergic neurotransmission.
In one study, [^{11}C]doxepin was used to see whether human depression depends on histaminergic mechanisms (Kano et al. 2004). The binding potential of the PET radioligand in some brain regions was lower in depressed patients than in healthy subjects and was correlated negatively to the patient's self-rated depression severity. In another PET study, the role of cholinergic processes in major depressive disorder was studied using [^{18}F]FP-TZTP (Cannon et al. 2006a). The depressed patients had a diagnosis of either recurrent major depressive disorder or bipolar disorder. [^{18}F]FP-TZTP binding in cortical brain regions and white matter was lower in bipolar depressed patients than in healthy subjects and was correlated negatively to depression severity. A third PET study used 2-[^{18}F]FA-85380 to look at cholinergic function and self-rated symptoms of depression in patients with Parkinson disease (Meyer et al. 2009b). Although none of the Parkinson patients met standard criteria for major depressive disorder (Schrag et al. 2007;Bech 1984), negative correlations were noted between self-rated depression scores and binding of the PET radiotracer in several cortical regions. Another PET study of subjects with only mild self-rated symptoms of depression used [^{18}F]FDDNP to explore possible correlations with aggregates of amyloid and tau proteins in brain regions (Lavretsky et al. 2009). Subjects with mild cognitive impairment showed a positive correlation between self-rated depression scores and radioligand binding in medial temporal lobe.

7. Challenges for PET neuroimaging of depressive disorders

Molecular tools currently available for PET neuroimaging in humans assess primarily monoaminergic receptors on surface of brain cells. As a result, most PET neuroimaging studies of depressive disorder focus on some aspect of the monoamine hypothesis. In our view, such PET studies have neither proved nor refuted conclusively any aspect of the monoamine hypothesis for depression (Schildkraut and Kety 1967;Asberg et al. 1976;Meltzer and Lowy 1987). While that monoamine hypothesis has been fruitful in certain ways, advances in neurobiology and neuropsychopharmacology have introduced a variety of additional molecular mechanisms into research on depressive disorders (Figure 1). Today, depression is viewed as the result of multiple neurobiological processes including disturbances of gene expression, intracellular signaling, cytokines and neurotropic agents (Tanis and Duman 2007;Berton and Nestler 2006;Krishnan and Nestler 2008;Maes 2008;Pittenger and Duman 2008). In our view, the success of PET scanning in determining the role of diverse neurobiological processes in depression will depend heavily on the invention of appropriate molecular tools, in the form of positron-emitting radioligands, for testing directly, in the living human brain, ever-changing hypotheses on causal connections between neuromolecular processes and the symptoms and severity of depressive disorders.

PET neuroimaging has been unable to pinpoint neurobiological defects in the brain of humans suffering from depressive disorders. This is perhaps not surprising, given the limited number of suitable positron-emitting radioligands that are currently available for PET studies of neurobiological processes in humans. Despite more than two decades of research, inconsistent findings have been obtained between molecular PET studies of depressive disorders, with few replication attempts. An important challenge facing PET neuroimaging of depressive disorders resides, therefore, in determining which aspects of depressive disorders to study next. We propose that particular attention be given to studying antidepressant non-response by PET, because that condition remains a major challenge for medical and social resources, with 25 – 50% of people suffering from major depressive disorder never recovering fully (Rush et al. 2003b;Rush et al. 2008;Fava 2003;Petersen et al. 2005;Berlim and Turecki 2007). Severe aberrations in molecular mechanisms at multiple cerebral sites may be involved in antidepressant non-response (Krishnan and Nestler 2008;Berton and Nestler 2006;Ressler and Mayberg 2007;Drevets et al. 2008). Success in determining by PET the neurobiological basis of antidepressant non-response can be expected to provide an improved understanding of depressive disorders and point to more effective ways of treating them.

The richness of human emotions, thoughts, and actions along with the complexity of molecular events in the human brain caution, however, against expectations of rapid progress in discovering by PET neuroimaging an improved diagnostic system or a panacea for depression (MacQueen 2009). This brings us to another challenge for PET neuroimaging of depressive disorders, namely that of integrating rapid advances in neuroscience into suitable positron-emitting radioligands and PET research designs. In view of the heterogeneous nature of depressive disorders (Berlim and Turecki 2007;Parker 2000;Pae et al. 2009;Thase 2009), multiple molecular pathways may cause symptoms of the disease. Some of the pathways that may be causally connected to depressive disorders include genes that encode presynaptic vesicular proteins, plasma membrane receptors, intracellular signaling molecules, proteins that regulate the actin cytoskeleton, and the transcriptional regulatory machinery (Covington, III et al. 2010). Additional molecular pathways thought to be either causative or curative of depression include neuroplasticity, neuropeptides, and nitric oxide synthase (Pittenger and Duman 2008;Paschos et al. 2009;Wegener and Volke 2010). Clearly, responding promptly to ever-changing notions on molecular pathways of depressive disorders constitutes a major challenge for PET neuroimaging.

Another challenging issue for PET neuroimaging of depressive disorders concerns financial support of research. Compared with the costs of brain diseases in the US and Europe

(Sobocki et al. 2006;Greenberg et al. 2003;Russell et al. 2004), national funding of molecular brain imaging is miniscule. In Europe, for example, the total annual cost of depression in 2004 was 120 billion Euro, for a population of 466 million with at least 21 million affected residents (Sobocki et al. 2006), making depression the most costly brain disorder. In contrast, recent annual funding for molecular brain imaging of depressive disorders can be estimated at only 0.001 - 0.003 billion Euro, which is 100,000 times less than the annual cost of the disease. Without substantial funding, molecular brain imaging by PET may continue to be severely handicapped in providing reliable findings on molecular causes, consequences, and cures of depressive disorders.

An additional challenge for PET neuroimaging of depressive disorders concerns the invention of appropriate research strategies for testing multiple hypotheses on molecular mechanisms in the living brain. At present, two opposing strategies characterize research in this field. One strategy advocates the use of positron-emitting radioligands with marked selectivity and high affinity for a single, specific neuronal macromolecule such as a monoamine receptor or enzyme. That approach has, in fact, been used in the majority of PET studies on molecular mechanisms in depression and may reflect the assumption that depressive disorders are caused by a dysfunction of a single molecular mechanism. The other strategy advocates the use of positron-emitting radioligands with affinities for several neuronal macromolecules. This approach may rest on the assumption that depressive disorders are caused by disturbances in any number of multiple molecular pathways. Recently, we followed the notion of multiple molecular pathways in a PET study of treatment-resistant depression (Smith et al. 2009). Using [^{11}C]mirtazapine, a positron-emitting radioligand of an antidepressant drug affecting several receptor systems (Millan 2006;Millan 2009;Smith et al. 2007), we studied by PET a group of depressed subjects who had failed to benefit from at least two antidepressant treatments (Smith et al. 2009). All subjects had received no antidepressant medication for at least 2 months before the study. We found that binding potentials of [^{11}C]mirtazapine in cerebral cortical regions were, in general, lower in depressed nonresponders than in healthy controls, while removal rates of [^{11}C]mirtazapine were generally higher in diencephalic regions of depressed nonresponders than in healthy controls. In keeping with the notion that depressive disorders are heterogeneous (Berlim and Turecki 2007;Parker 2000;Pae et al. 2009;Thase 2009), we noted that the binding of [^{11}C]mirtazapine in brain regions of some of the depressed, antidepressant-nonresponders was well-within the normal range, whereas reduced regional binding of [^{11}C]mirtazapine was noted in other depressed subjects. A challenge for additional PET studies with [^{11}C]mirtazapine is to see whether the procedure can provide a neuromolecular-screening devise that can distinguish between neurobiologically-distinct subgroups of depressed, antidepressant-nonresponders.

One of the most formidable challenges for PET neuroimaging of depressive disorders relates to the blood-brain-barrier (BBB). The BBB is a limiting factor for PET studies of neuromolecular processes in the living human brain because it both restricts the passage of endogenous and foreign substances into the brain and expels many substances rapidly from the brain (Beduneau et al. 2008;Gjedde et al. 2000;Halldin et al. 2001;Kreuter 2001;Laruelle et al. 2002;Misra et al. 2003;Tosi et al. 2008). Thus, failure to traverse the BBB in sufficient quantities and/or to remain in brain tissue for a sufficient duration in the course of a PET-scanning session has caused many candidate radioligands to be discarded. PET neuroscientists will need to devise ways of improving the passage of novel positron-emitting radioligands across the BBB for binding to molecular targets within the central nervous system. One possibility that may deserve close attention in the time ahead concerns the use of nanoparticles in PET neuroimaging. Some nanoparticles have already been shown to markedly enhance the level of certain drugs in the central nervous system (Gelperina et al. 2009;Kreuter 2002;Vergoni et al. 2009), indicating a potential role of nanoparticles as carrier-molecules for ushering novel PET radioligands to their neurobiological targets.

8. Challenges for PET radiochemistry

The synthesis and development of radiopharmaceuticals for PET is a complicated and extremely challenging process. The main challenge of using the short-lived PET radioisotopes carbon-11 ($t_{1/2}$ = 20.4 min), fluorine-18 ($t_{1/2}$ = 110 min), nitrogen-13 ($t_{1/2}$ = 9.97 min) or oxygen-15 ($t_{1/2}$ = 2.04 min) for the synthesis of radiopharmaceuticals is that of time (Fowler and Wolf 1997). The short half-lives of these radioisotopes imposes severe time restrictions when preparing radiolabelled compounds for PET. Such short time periods limit the range of synthetic strategies that are available to obtain target radiolabelled compounds, confining them to chemical reactions and processes that are on the order of seconds and minutes rather than hours. Many PET radiolabelling procedures are therefore limited to only one or two distinct chemical steps with the introduction of the PET radioisotope as late in the radiosynthesis as possible. The radioisotopes ^{13}N and ^{15}O are of limited applicability for imaging receptor-related processes of the CNS because their short half-lives prohibit the synthesis of complex tracer molecules and are generally not commensurate with the time frames required for monitoring ligand-receptor based processes. ^{11}C and ^{18}F are therefore the most commonly used radioisotopes in PET for imaging neuroreceptor processes, having half-lives that are long enough to enable multi-step synthesis of quite complex radioligands in addition to being appropriate for monitoring ligand-receptor processes. The choice of which radioisotope, ^{11}C or ^{18}F, to use depends on a number of decisive factors. Firstly, the structure of the target molecule. For example, does it have fluorine atom and would introducing an ^{18}F adversely affect its biological properties? Secondly, the ease of synthesis. Can the target molecule be synthesised using available chemical techniques and are the appropriate ^{18}F or ^{11}C precursors available for reaction? There may be an obvious advantage in using one radioisotope over the other in terms of radiochemical yield, specific activity or speed of labelling. Thirdly, the time frame of the biological process under investigation; ^{18}F may be a more appropriate isotope for the investigation of longer biological processes such as protein synthesis.

Carbon is present in all natural products and almost every artificially synthesised drug-like compound. The replacement of a naturally abundant ^{12}C atom with that of a positron-emitting ^{11}C isotope results in ^{11}C-labeled molecules that will have essentially identical chemical and biological properties of the parent compound. This is a hugely important feature since it removes any doubts about the effect of introducing an artificial exogenous radioisotope (e.g. ^{18}F) or tag (e.g. [Ga-DOTA] complex) into the parent molecule which may affect its biological behaviour. Although the short 20 min half-life of ^{11}C precludes long multistep syntheses, a wide range of chemical reactions have been developed for synthesising ^{11}C labelled compounds (Miller et al. 2008). In comparison, ^{18}F has a considerably longer half-life of 110 min which permits longer and more complex radiosynthetic strategies in addition to allowing the transportation of doses to scanning sites several hours away. The key concern, alluded to above, of introducing an ^{18}F radioisotope into a molecule is the unknown effects the fluorine atom may have on the biological properties of the newly labelled compound. Radiosynthesis with ^{18}F may be classified into two areas: (i) direct fluorination, where the ^{18}F isotope is introduced into the target molecule in one chemical step, and (ii) indirect fluorination which requires a multi-step synthesis for the preparation of so-called ^{18}F prosthetic groups that are then further reacted to give the target molecule. Considerable effort has been devoted to the development of these small and reactive ^{18}F prosthetic groups for the rapid labelling of a range of ^{18}F molecules. In recent years the development of rapid 'click chemistry' methods continues to generate much interest in this area (Glaser and Robins 2009).

Some of the challenges within PET radiochemistry are evidently more obvious than others and relate to the technical challenges associated with the fast, efficient and safe handling of short-lived radioactive material. The production of a pharmaceutical-quality radiotracer sample ready for injection requires the synthesis, purification, and analysis to be complete, generally, within three half-lives of the radioisotope in order to provide enough radioactivity for a reliable scan. In the case of a ^{11}C radiosynthesis, this would be within 60 min from the end of bombardment. The need for such fast reactions and processes has lead, not only to new chemical methodologies, but to technological advancements in the development of fully automated and programmable synthesis units for performing and processing radiosynthetic reactions. New technologies such as microwave cavities (Elander et al. 2000), microfluidic reactors (Miller 2009), and solid-phase synthesis methods (Marik et al. 2006) have been adapted to enhance the speed, reproducibility, and efficiency of radiolabelling reactions.

Other challenges are more subtle and include the unusual scale of PET labelling reactions where the cold precursor in the reaction is often in huge excess (>1000 fold) compared with the radiolabelled compound. This can lead to unpredictable reaction kinetics and the formation of unwanted by-products from competing side reactions. There is often a desire to improve radiochemical yields (RCY) and to obtain high specific activities from labelling reactions. Although high RCYs are not always essential, they do provide a very useful measure of the efficiency of the radiolabelling procedure. The requirement of high specific activity, on the other hand, is often essential for the study of neuroreceptors such as those associated with depressive disorders. Specific activities of a radiolabelled compound for a PET study of neuroreceptors are typically required to be in the order of 50–500 GBq μmol^{-1}.

The requirement of high specific activities is most apparent if the radioligand has a high affinity for a receptor. Radiotracers produced with low specific activity will result in poor PET images owing to the rapid saturation of the binding sites by the proportionately higher amount of non-radioactive ligand. The production of radiotracers with high specific activity is therefore highly desirable but can be challenging and depends on the radioisotope selected for the radiosynthesis, choice of synthetic precursor material and radiosynthetic labelling route. Take, for example, the selective 5-HT_{1A} receptor antagonist WAY-100635 which can be radiolabelled using ^{11}C in the carbonyl position to give [*carbonyl*-^{11}C]WAY-100635 (figure 2). This is usually achieved via the two-step reaction of $^{11}CO_2$ with cyclohexylmagnesium chloride sequentially followed by addition of thionyl chloride to give the reactive [*carbonyl*-^{11}C]cyclohexyl acid chloride. Reaction of [*carbonyl*-^{11}C]cyclohexyl acid chloride with the WAY-100634 amine precursor generates the desired [*carbonyl*-^{11}C]WAY-100635 (McCarron et al. 1996). One of the key challenges with the synthesis of [*carbonyl*-

^{11}C]WAY-100635 is the exclusion of atmospheric $^{12}CO_2$ which poses a significant risk of contaminating the reaction at the initial first step. Without due care, contamination from atmospheric ^{12}C results in an undesirably low specific radioactivity, and consequently poor PET images.

The labelling position of radioisotope on the ligand is also a key consideration, and can pose significant challenges. Two key questions should be asked regarding labelling position, (i) is it viable, synthetically, to radiolabel in the position that we desire? and (ii) will the labelling position be metabolically stable? An understanding of the metabolic fate of a radiotracer can be vitally important in the development of a radiotracer and in determining the best position to radiolabel. There is usually a choice of positions within the molecule for radioisotope labelling, with some positions being more challenging than others. However, labelling a molecule in several different positions can yield important metabolic information about the fate of the molecule *in vivo* and can be useful in determining which labelling position is best for imaging. Metabolism of the labelled compound in the body may result in undesired labelled metabolites which can give two undesired effects: (i) an enhanced unwanted background signal which results in poor quality PET image, and (ii) pharmacologically active metabolites that compete with the parent compound for the biological target and complicate the interpretation of PET data. The importance of the labelling position can be illustrated by past experiences with the ^{11}C labelling of WAY-100635 radioligand. WAY-100635 can be labelled in either the *O*-methyl position on the phenyl ring via a [^{11}C]methylation reaction or on the carbonyl position as previously mentioned above (figure 2). [*O-methyl*-^{11}C]WAY-100635 was however found to have limitations for imaging 5-HT$_{1A}$ receptors in human owing to the formation of the more lipophilic descyclohexanecarbonyl ([*O-methyl*-^{11}C]WAY-100634) metabolite *in vivo*. This metabolite was found to enter the brain much more readily than the parent [*O-methyl*-^{11}C]WAY-100635 (Osman et al. 1996) and thus complicate quantification of the 5-HT$_{1A}$ receptors by competing with [*O-methyl*-^{11}C]WAY-100635 for 5-HT$_{1A}$ binding sites and by contributing to the non-specific binding signal. In contrast, by selecting to label WAY-100635 in the carbonyl position (figure 2) significantly improved PET images with much superior delineation of 5-HT$_{1A}$ receptors in human brain were obtained (Pike et al. 1996). The reason for [*carbonyl*-^{11}C]WAY-100635 giving better images is due to the metabolism of this compound and position of the radioisotope; with the ^{11}C isotope on the carbonyl group adjacent to the cyclohexyl ring, *in vivo* metabolism cleaves the cyclohexyl and ^{11}C carbonyl and generates the labelled metabolite [^{11}C]cyclohexanecarboxylic acid which is hydrophilic and, therefore, does not readily enter the brain to confound the signal from the parent [*carbonyl*-^{11}C]WAY-100635 molecule.

Appropriate pharmacodynamic properties, such as high affinities and selectivities for the target, are central to characterising the success of a PET radioligand (Passchier et al. 2002). The affinity of the probe for the binding site is a key factor that affects the degree of nonspecific binding. Nonspecific binding is a major challenge in the development of radioligands and is often cited for the high failure rate of new radioligands. Nonspecific binding occurs when the radioligand binds or interacts with a molecular target or tissue other than the site of interest. This could include interactions of the radioligand with membrane structures or with receptors which are not under investigation. A high proportion of nonspecific binding signal may result in a severe reduction in the PET signal contrast when investigating a specific receptor with a radioligand. The lipophilicity of the tracer molecule is frequently quoted as an important factor in discussions of nonspecific binding. Highly lipophilic molecules are known to interact extensively with the fatty residues in membrane bilayers which can prevent penetration of the radioligand into brain tissue and therefore prevent it from reaching the intended molecular target. The challenges in terms of the design and selection of tracer molecules to image the CNS often involve tailoring the lipophilicity of a radioligand. Successful PET CNS radiotracers normally have lipophilicities (logP, logarithm of the octanol/water partition coefficient) within an optimal logP window of 1.5-3 in order to ensure the passage through the BBB. Although logP values are an important indicator in ligand design, they can lead to an oversimplification of ligand selection. A greater understanding of the causes of nonspecific binding at a molecular level may be key to achieving higher success rates for radioligand selection. A recent study has used computation methods to estimate the interaction energy between candidate molecules and phospholipids which can then be used as a predictor for nonspecific binding *in vivo* (Rosso et al. 2008). Results from this study interestingly show that the drug's interaction with the lipid molecule is a better predictor for nonspecific binding than the experimentally measured logP value. Further recent work in this area suggests that alternative transport mechanisms of drug molecules through biological membranes, which result in the chemically activated degradation of the phospholipid membranes, may be related to nonspecific binding (Casey et al. 2008).

Concluding remark

We hope that the challenges described here will inspire scientists to carry out many more studies using PET neuroimaging in order to eventually discover new and better procedures for diagnosing and treating major depressive disorders.

9. Chemical names

Altanserin	3-2-4-4-Fluorobenzoyl-1-piperidinylethyl-2,3-dihydro-2-thioxo-41*H*-quinazolinone
DASB	3-Amino-4-[[2-[dimethylaminomethyl] phenyl]thio] benzonitrile
DOTA	1,4,7,10-tetraazacyclododecane-1,4,7,10-tetraacetic acid
Doxepin	3-dibenzo[*b,e*]oxepin-116*H*-ylidene-*N,N*-dimethylpropan-1-amine
2-FA-85380	2-fluoro-3-(2[S]-2-azetidinylmethoxy)-pyridine
FCWAY	*N*-[2-[4-2-Methoxyphenyl-1-piperazinyl]ethyl]-*N*-2-pyridinyl-*trans*-4-fluorocyclohexylcarboxamide
FDDNP	2-(1-{6-_(2-_fluorine-18_fluoroethyl)(methyl)amino-2-naphthyl}ethylidene) malononitrile
FESP	3-2-Fluoroethyl-8-[4-4-fluorophenyl-4-oxobutyl]-1-phenyl-1,3,8-triazaspiro[4.5]decan-4-one
FLB 457	5-Bromo-*N*-[[2*S*-1-ethyl-2-pyrrolidinyl]methyl]-2,3-dimethoxybenzamide
Fluoro-L-dopa	2-Fluoro-5-hydroxy-L-tyrosine
FP-TZTP	3-3-3-Flouropropylthio-1,2,5-thiadiazol-4-yl-1,2,5,6-tetrahydro-1-methylpyridine

Harmine	7-Methoxy-1-methyl-9*H*-[3,4-*b*]indole
McNeil 5652	6*S*,10b*R*-1,2,3,5,6,10b-Hexahydro-6-[4-methylthiophenyl]-pyrrolo[2,1-a]isoquinoline
MDL 100,907	*R*-1-[2-4-Fluorophenylethyl]-4-2,3-dimethoxyphenyl-4-piperidinemethano
MPPF	4-Fluoro-*N*-[2-[4-2-methoxyphenyl-1-piperazinyl]ethyl]-*N*-2-pyridinylbenzamide
α-MTrp	α-Methyl-L-tryptophan
NNC-112	+-5-7-benzofuranyl-8-chloro-7-hydroxy-3-methyl-2,3,4,5-tetrahydro-1H-3-benzazapine
Raclopride	3,5-Dichloro-*N*-[[2*S*-1-ethyl-2-pyrrolidinyl]methyl]-2-hydroxy-6-methoxybenzamide
RTI-32	Methyl-1*R*-2-exo-3-exo-8-methyl-3-4-methylphenyl-8-azabicyclo[3.2.1]octane-2-carboxylate
SCH 23,390	8-Chloro-2,3,4,5-tetrahydro-3-methyl-5-phenyl-1*H*-3-benzazepin-7-ol
Setoperone	6-[2-[4-4-Fluorobenzoyl-1-piperidinyl]ethyl]-2,3-dihydro-7-methyl-5*H*-thiazolo[3,2a] pyrimidin-5-one
WAY-100635	*N*-[2-[4-2-Methoxyphenyl-1-piperazinyl]ethyl]-*N*-2-pyridinyl-cyclohexylcarboxamide

10. Conflict of interest

The authors declare that, except for income received from their primary employer, no financial support has been received for their research activity, including the writing of this review.

11. Acknowledgments

We thank everybody at the Center for Psychiatric Research and the PET Center of Aarhus University for providing a positive atmosphere in which to work. DFS thanks the Danish Medical Research Council for research funding, and PWM is grateful to the EPSRC for the award of a Life Sciences Interface fellowship (EP/E039278/1).

12. References

Asberg M, Thoren P, Traskman L, Bertilsson L, Ringberger V. 1976. "Serotonin depression"--a biochemical subgroup within the affective disorders? Science 191:478-480.

Bech P. 1984. The instrumental use of rating scales for depression. Pharmacopsychiatry 17:22-28.

Beduneau A, Hindre F, Clavreul A, Leroux JC, Saulnier P, Benoit JP. 2008. Brain targeting using novel lipid nanovectors. J Control Release 126:44-49.

Berlim MT, Fleck MP, Turecki G. 2008. Current trends in the assessment and somatic treatment of resistant/refractory major depression: an overview. Ann Med 40:149-159.

Berlim MT, Turecki G. 2007. What is the meaning of treatment resistant/refractory major depression (TRD)? A systematic review of current randomized trials. Eur Neuropsychopharmacol 17:696-707.

Berton O, Nestler EJ. 2006. New approaches to antidepressant drug discovery: beyond monoamines. Nat Rev Neurosci 7:137-151.

Bhagwagar Z, Hinz R, Taylor M, Fancy S, Cowen P, Grasby P. 2006. Increased 5-HT(2A) receptor binding in euthymic, medication-free patients recovered from depression: a positron emission study with [(11)C]MDL 100,907. Am J Psychiatry 163:1580-1587.

Bhagwagar Z, Murthy N, Selvaraj S, Hinz R, Taylor M, Fancy S, Grasby P, Cowen P. 2007. 5-HTT binding in recovered depressed patients and healthy volunteers: a positron emission tomography study with [11C]DASB. Am J Psychiatry 164:1858-1865.

Bhagwagar Z, Rabiner EA, Sargent PA, Grasby PM, Cowen PJ. 2004. Persistent reduction in brain serotonin1A receptor binding in recovered depressed men measured by positron emission tomography with [11C]WAY-100635. Mol Psychiatry 9:386-392.

Boileau I, Warsh JJ, Guttman M, Saint-Cyr JA, McCluskey T, Rusjan P, Houle S, Wilson AA, Meyer JH, Kish SJ. 2008. Elevated serotonin transporter binding in depressed patients with Parkinson's disease: a preliminary PET study with [11C]DASB. Mov Disord 23:1776-1780.

Bragulat V, Paillere-Martinot ML, Artiges E, Frouin V, Poline JB, Martinot JL. 2007. Dopaminergic function in depressed patients with affective flattening or with impulsivity: [18F]fluoro-L-dopa positron emission tomography study with voxel-based analysis. Psychiatry Res 154:115-124.

Busto UE, Redden L, Mayberg H, Kapur S, Houle S, Zawertailo LA. 2009. Dopaminergic activity in depressed smokers: a positron emission tomography study. Synapse 63:681-689.

Cannon DM, Carson RE, Nugent AC, Eckelman WC, Kiesewetter DO, Williams J, Rollis D, Drevets M, Gandhi S, Solorio G, Drevets WC. 2006a. Reduced muscarinic type 2 receptor binding in subjects with bipolar disorder. Arch Gen Psychiatry 63:741-747.

Cannon DM, Ichise M, Fromm SJ, Nugent AC, Rollis D, Gandhi SK, Klaver JM, Charney DS, Manji HK, Drevets WC. 2006b. Serotonin transporter binding in bipolar disorder assessed using [11C]DASB and positron emission tomography. Biol Psychiatry 60:207-217.

Cannon DM, Ichise M, Rollis D, Klaver JM, Gandhi SK, Charney DS, Manji HK, Drevets WC. 2007. Elevated serotonin transporter binding in major depressive disorder assessed using positron emission tomography and [11C]DASB; comparison with bipolar disorder. Biol Psychiatry 62:870-877.

Cannon DM, Klaver JM, Peck SA, Rallis-Voak D, Erickson K, Drevets WC. 2008. Dopamine Type-1 Receptor Binding in Major Depressive Disorder Assessed Using Positron Emission Tomography and [(11)C]NNC-112. Neuropsychopharmacology 34:1277-1287.

Casey DR, Sebai SC, Shearman GC, Ces O, Law RV, Templer RH, Gee AD. 2008. Formulation affects the rate of membrane degradation catalyzed by cationic amphiphilic drugs. Ind Eng Chem Res 47:650-655.

Covington HE, III, Vialou V, Nestler EJ. 2010. From synapse to nucleus: Novel targets for treating depression. Neuropharmacology 58:683-693.

Dougherty DD, Bonab AA, Ottowitz WE, Livni E, Alpert NM, Rauch SL, Fava M, Fischman AJ. 2006. Decreased striatal D1 binding as measured using PET and [11C]SCH 23,390 in patients with major depression with anger attacks. Depress Anxiety 23:175-177.

Drevets WC, Savitz J, Trimble M. 2008. The subgenual anterior cingulate cortex in mood disorders. CNS Spectr 13:663-681.

Drevets WC, Thase ME, Moses-Kolko EL, Price J, Frank E, Kupfer DJ, Mathis C. 2007. Serotonin-1A receptor imaging in recurrent depression: replication and literature review. Nucl Med Biol 34:865-877.

Dunlop BW, Nemeroff CB. 2007. The role of dopamine in the pathophysiology of depression. Arch Gen Psychiatry 64:327-337.

Elander N, Jones JR, Lu SY, Stone-Elander S. 2000. Microwave-enhanced radiochemistry. Chem Soc Rev 29:239-249.

Fava M. 2003. Diagnosis and definition of treatment-resistant depression. Biol Psychiatry 53:649-659.

Fowler JS, Wolf AP. 1997. Working against time: Rapid radiotracer synthesis and imaging the human brain. Accounts Chem Res 30:181-188.

Gelperina S, Maksimenko O, Khalansky A, Vanchugova L, Shipulo E, Abbasova K, Berdiev R, Wohlfart S, Chepurnova N, Kreuter J. 2010. Drug delivery to the brain using surfactant-coated poly(lactide-co-glycolide) nanoparticles: Influence of the formulation parameters. Eur J Pharm Biopharm 74:157-163.

Gjedde A, Gee AD, Smith DF. 2000. Basic CNS Drug Transport and Binding Kinetics in Vivo. In: Begley DJ, Bradbury MW, Kreuter J, editors. The Blood-Brain Barrier and Drug Delivery to the CNS2. New York / Basel: Marcel Dekker, Inc.p 225-243.

Glaser M, Robins EG. 2009. 'Click labelling' in PET radiochemistry. J Label Compd Radiopharm 52:407-414.

Greenberg PE, Kessler RC, Birnbaum HG, Leong SA, Lowe SW, Berglund PA, Corey-Lisle PK. 2003. The economic burden of depression in the United States: how did it change between 1990 and 2000? J Clin Psychiatry 64:1465-1475.

Halldin C, Gulyas B, Langer O, Farde L. 2001. Brain radioligands--state of the art and new trends. Q J Nucl Med 45:139-152.

Hindmarch I. 2002. Beyond the monoamine hypothesis: mechanisms, molecules and methods. Eur Psychiatry 17 Suppl 3:294-299.

Hirvonen J, Karlsson H, Kajander J, Lepola A, Markkula J, Rasi-Hakala H, Nagren K, Salminen JK, Hietala J. 2008. Decreased brain serotonin 5-HT1A receptor availability in medication-naive patients with major depressive disorder: an in-vivo imaging study using PET and [carbonyl-11C]WAY-100635. Int J Neuropsychopharmacol 11:465-476.

Kano M, Fukudo S, Tashiro A, Utsumi A, Tamura D, Itoh M, Iwata R, Tashiro M, Mochizuki H, Funaki Y, Kato M, Hongo M, Yanai K. 2004. Decreased histamine H1 receptor binding in the brain of depressed patients. Eur J Neurosci 20:803-810.

Kreuter J. 2001. Nanoparticulate systems for brain delivery of drugs. Adv Drug Deliv Rev 47:65-81.

Kreuter J. 2002. Transport of drugs across the blood-brain barrier by nanoparticles. Curr Med Chem - Centr Nerv Syst Agents 2:241-249.

Krishnan V, Nestler EJ. 2008. The molecular neurobiology of depression. Nature 455:894-902.

Kuroda Y, Motohashi N, Ito H, Ito S, Takano A, Nishikawa T, Suhara T. 2006. Effects of repetitive transcranial magnetic stimulation on [11C]raclopride binding and cognitive function in patients with depression. J Affect Disord 95:35-42.

Lammertsma AA. 2002. Radioligand studies: imaging and quantitative analysis. Eur Neuropsychopharmacol 12:513-516.

Laruelle M. 2000. Imaging synaptic neurotransmission with in vivo binding competition techniques: a critical review. J Cereb Blood Flow Metab 20:423-451.

Laruelle M, Slifstein M, Huang Y. 2002. Positron emission tomography: imaging and quantification of neurotransporter availability. Methods 27:287-299.

Lavretsky H, Siddarth P, Kepe V, Ercoli LM, Miller KJ, Burggren AC, Bookheimer SY, Huang SC, Barrio JR, Small GW. 2009. Depression and anxiety symptoms are associated with cerebral FDDNP-PET binding in middle-aged and older nondemented adults. Am J Geriatr Psychiatry 17:493-502.

MacQueen GM. 2009. Magnetic resonance imaging and prediction of outcome in patients with major depressive disorder. J Psychiatry Neurosci 34:343-349.

Maes M. 2008. The cytokine hypothesis of depression: inflammation, oxidative & nitrosative stress (IO&NS) and leaky gut as new targets for adjunctive treatments in depression. Neuro Endocrinol Lett 29:287-291.

Marik J, Hausner SH, Fix LA, Gagnon MKJ, Sutcliffe JL. 2006. Solid-phase synthesis of 2-[F-18]fluoropropionyl peptides. Bioconjugate Chem. 17:1017-1021.

McCarron JA, Turton DR, Pike VW, Poole KG. 1996. Remotely-controlled production of the 5-HT1A receptor radioligand, [carbonyl-C-11]WAY-100635, via C-11-carboxylation of an immobilized Grignard reagent. J Label Compd Radiopharm 38:941-953.

Meltzer CC, Price JC, Mathis CA, Butters MA, Ziolko SK, Moses-Kolko E, Mazumdar S, Mulsant BH, Houck PR, Lopresti BJ, Weissfeld LA, Reynolds CF. 2004. Serotonin 1A receptor binding and treatment response in late-life depression. Neuropsychopharmacology 29:2258-2265.

Meltzer HY, Lowy MT. 1987. The serotonin hypothesis of depression. In: Meltzer HY, editor. Psychopharmacology: The Third Generation of Progress. New York: Raven Press. p 513-526.

Meyer JH, Ginovart N, Boovariwala A, Sagrati S, Hussey D, Garcia A, Young T, Praschak-Rieder N, Wilson AA, Houle S. 2006a. Elevated monoamine oxidase a levels in the brain: an explanation for the monoamine imbalance of major depression. Arch Gen Psychiatry 63:1209-1216.

Meyer JH, Houle S, Sagrati S, Carella A, Hussey DF, Ginovart N, Goulding V, Kennedy J, Wilson AA. 2004. Brain serotonin transporter binding potential measured with carbon 11-labeled DASB positron emission tomography: effects of major depressive episodes and severity of dysfunctional attitudes. Arch Gen Psychiatry 61:1271-1279.

Meyer JH, McMain S, Kennedy SH, Korman L, Brown GM, DaSilva JN, Wilson AA, Blak T, Eynan-Harvey R, Goulding VS, Houle S, Links P. 2003. Dysfunctional attitudes and 5-HT2 receptors during depression and self-harm. Am J Psychiatry 160:90-99.

Meyer JH, McNeely HE, Sagrati S, Boovariwala A, Martin K, Verhoeff NP, Wilson AA, Houle S. 2006b. Elevated putamen D(2) receptor binding potential in major depression with motor retardation: an [11C]raclopride positron emission tomography study. Am J Psychiatry 163:1594-1602.

Meyer JH, Wilson AA, Sagrati S, Miler L, Rusjan P, Bloomfield PM, Clark M, Sacher J, Voineskos AN, Houle S. 2009a. Brain monoamine oxidase A binding in major depressive disorder: relationship to selective serotonin reuptake inhibitor treatment, recovery, and recurrence. Arch Gen Psychiatry 66:1304-1312.

Meyer PM, Strecker K, Kendziorra K, Becker G, Hesse S, Woelpl D, Hensel A, Patt M, Sorger D, Wegner F, Lobsien D, Barthel H, Brust P, Gertz HJ, Sabri O, Schwarz J. 2009b. Reduced alpha4beta2*-nicotinic acetylcholine receptor binding and its relationship to mild cognitive and depressive symptoms in Parkinson disease. Arch Gen Psychiatry 66:866-877.

Mickey BJ, Ducci F, Hodgkinson CA, Langenecker SA, Goldman D, Zubieta JK. 2008. Monoamine oxidase A genotype predicts human serotonin 1A receptor availability in vivo. J Neurosci 28:11354-11359.

Millan MJ. 2006. Multi-target strategies for the improved treatment of depressive states: Conceptual foundations and neuronal substrates, drug discovery and therapeutic application. Pharmacol Ther 110:135-370.

Millan MJ. 2009. Dual- and triple-acting agents for treating core and co-morbid symptoms of major depression: novel concepts, new drugs. Neurotherapeutics 6:53-77.

Miller JM, Brennan KG, Ogden TR, Oquendo MA, Sullivan GM, Mann JJ, Parsey RV. 2009a. Elevated serotonin 1A binding in remitted major depressive disorder: evidence for a trait biological abnormality. Neuropsychopharmacology 34:2275-2284.

Miller JM, Kinnally EL, Ogden RT, Oquendo MA, Mann JJ, Parsey RV. 2009b. Reported childhood abuse is associated with low serotonin transporter binding in vivo in major depressive disorder. Synapse 63:565-573.

Miller JM, Oquendo MA, Ogden RT, Mann JJ, Parsey RV. 2008. Serotonin transporter binding as a possible predictor of one-year remission in major depressive disorder. J Psychiatr Res 42:1137-1142.

Miller PW. 2009. Radiolabelling with short-lived PET (positron emission tomography) isotopes using microfluidic reactors. J Chem Technol Biotechnol 84:309-315.

Miller PW, Long NJ, Vilar R, Gee AD. 2008. Synthesis of C-11, F-18, O-15, and N-13 Radiolabels for Positron Emission Tomography. Angew Chem Int Edit 47:8998-9033.

Mintun MA, Sheline YI, Moerlein SM, Vlassenko AG, Huang Y, Snyder AZ. 2004. Decreased hippocampal 5-HT2A receptor binding in major depressive disorder: in vivo measurement with [18F]altanserin positron emission tomography. Biol Psychiatry 55:217-224.

Misra A, Ganesh S, Shahiwala A, Shah SP. 2003. Drug delivery to the central nervous system: a review. J Pharm Pharm Sci 6:252-273.

Montgomery AJ, Stokes P, Kitamura Y, Grasby PM. 2007. Extrastriatal D2 and striatal D2 receptors in depressive illness: pilot PET studies using [11C]FLB 457 and [11C]raclopride. J Affect Disord 101:113-122.

Moses-Kolko EL, Price JC, Thase ME, Meltzer CC, Kupfer DJ, Mathis CA, Bogers WD, Berman SR, Houck PR, Schneider TN, Drevets WC. 2007. Measurement of 5-HT1A receptor binding in depressed adults before and after antidepressant drug treatment using positron emission tomography and [11C]WAY-100635. Synapse 61:523-530.

Nemeroff CB, Owens MJ. 2009. The role of serotonin in the pathophysiology of depression: as important as ever. Clin Chem 55:1578-1579.

Oquendo MA, Hastings RS, Huang YY, Simpson N, Ogden RT, Hu XZ, Goldman D, Arango V, van Heertum RL, Mann JJ, Parsey RV. 2007. Brain serotonin transporter binding in depressed patients with bipolar disorder using positron emission tomography. Arch Gen Psychiatry 64:201-208.

Osman S, Lundkvist C, Pike VW, Halldin C, McCarron JA, Swahn CG, Ginovart N, Luthra SK, Bench CJ, Grasby PM, Wikstrom H, Barf T, Cliffe IA, Fletcher A, Farde L. 1996. Characterization of the radioactive metabolites of the 5-HT1A receptor radioligand, [O-methyl-C-11]WAY-100635, in monkey and human plasma by HPLC: Comparison of the behaviour of an identified radioactive metabolite with parent radioligand in monkey using PET. Nucl Med Biol 23:627-634.

Owens MJ, Nemeroff CB. 1994. Role of serotonin in the pathophysiology of depression: focus on the serotonin transporter. Clin Chem 40:288-295.

Pae CU, Tharwani H, Marks DM, Masand PS, Patkar AA. 2009. Atypical depression: a comprehensive review. CNS Drugs 23:1023-1037.

Parker G. 2000. Classifying depression: should paradigms lost be regained? Am J Psychiatry 157:1195-1203.

Parsey RV, Hastings RS, Oquendo MA, Huang YY, Simpson N, Arcement J, Huang Y, Ogden RT, van Heertum RL, Arango V, Mann JJ. 2006a. Lower serotonin transporter binding potential in the human brain during major depressive episodes. Am J Psychiatry 163:52-58.

Parsey RV, Oquendo MA, Ogden RT, Olvet DM, Simpson N, Huang YY, van Heertum RL, Arango V, Mann JJ. 2006b. Altered serotonin 1A binding in major depression: a [carbonyl-C-11]WAY100635 positron emission tomography study. Biol Psychiatry 59:106-113.

Paschos KA, Veletza S, Chatzaki E. 2009. Neuropeptide and sigma receptors as novel therapeutic targets for the pharmacotherapy of depression. CNS Drugs 23:755-772.

Passchier J, Gee A, Willemsen A, Vaalburg W, van Waarde A. 2002. Measuring drug-related receptor occupancy with positron emission tomography. Methods 27:278-286

Petersen T, Papakostas GI, Posternak MA, Kant A, Guyker WM, Iosifescu DV, Yeung AS, Nierenberg AA, Fava M. 2005. Empirical testing of two models for staging antidepressant treatment resistance. J Clin Psychopharmacol 25:336-341.

Pike VW, McCarron JA, Lammertsma AA, Osman S, Hume SP, Sargent PA, Bench CJ, Cliffe IA, Fletcher A, Grasby PM. 1996. Exquisite delineation of 5-HT1A receptors in human brain with PET and [carbonyl-C-11]WAY-100635. Eur J Pharmacol 301:R5-R7.

Pittenger C, Duman RS. 2008. Stress, depression, and neuroplasticity: a convergence of mechanisms. Neuropsychopharmacology 33:88-109.

Praschak-Rieder N, Hussey D, Wilson AA, Carella A, Lee M, Dunn E, Willeit M, Bagby RM, Houle S, Meyer JH. 2004. Tryptophan depletion and serotonin loss in selective serotonin reuptake inhibitor-treated depression: an [(18)F] MPPF positron emission tomography study. Biol Psychiatry 56:587-591.

Randrup A, Braestrup C. 1977. Uptake inhibition of biogenic amines by newer antidepressant drugs: relevance to the dopamine hypothesis of depression. Psychopharmacology (Berl) 53:309-314.

Reimold M, Batra A, Knobel A, Smolka MN, Zimmer A, Mann K, Solbach C, Reischl G, Schwarzler F, Grunder G, Machulla HJ, Bares R, Heinz A. 2008. Anxiety is associated with reduced central serotonin transporter availability in unmedicated patients with unipolar major depression: a [11C]DASB PET study. Mol Psychiatry 13:606-613.

Reivich M, Amsterdam JD, Brunswick DJ, Shiue CY. 2004. PET brain imaging with [11C](+)McN5652 shows increased serotonin transporter availability in major depression. J Affect Disord 82:321-327.

Remy P, Doder M, Lees A, Turjanski N, Brooks D. 2005. Depression in Parkinson's disease: loss of dopamine and noradrenaline innervation in the limbic system. Brain 128:1314-1322.
Ressler KJ, Mayberg HS. 2007. Targeting abnormal neural circuits in mood and anxiety disorders: from the laboratory to the clinic. Nat Neurosci 10:1116 1124.
Rosso L, Gee AD, Gould IR. 2008. Ab initio computational study of positron emission tomography ligands interacting with lipid molecule for the prediction of nonspecific binding. J Comput Chem 29:2397-2405.
Rush AJ, Thase ME, Dube S. 2003a. Research issues in the study of difficult-to-treat depression. Biol Psychiatry 53:743-753.
Rush AJ, Warden D, Wisniewski SR, Fava M, Trivedi MH, Gaynes BN, Nierenberg AA. 2009. STAR*D: Revising Conventional Wisdom. CNS Drugs 23:627-647.
Rush AJ, Wisniewski SR, Warden D, Luther JF, Davis LL, Fava M, Nierenberg AA, Trivedi MH. 2008. Selecting among second-step antidepressant medication monotherapies: predictive value of clinical, demographic, or first-step treatment features. Arch Gen Psychiatry 65:870-880.
Russell JM, Hawkins K, Ozminkowski RJ, Orsini L, Crown WH, Kennedy S, Finkelstein S, Berndt E, Rush AJ. 2004. The cost consequences of treatment-resistant depression. J Clin Psychiatry 65:341-347.
Saijo T, Takano A, Suhara T, Arakawa R, Okumura M, Ichimiya T, Ito H, Okubo Y. 2010. Effect of electroconvulsive therapy on 5-HT1A receptor binding in patients with depression: a PET study with [11C]WAY 100635. Int J Neuropsychopharmacol 13:785-791.
Schildkraut JJ, Davis JM, Klerman GL. 1968. Biochemistry of Depressions. Psychopharmacology: A Review of Progress, 1957-1967. Bethesda, Maryland: National Institute of Mental Health. P. 625-648.
Schildkraut JJ, Kety SS. 1967. Biogenic amines and emotion. Science 156:21-30.
Schrag A, Barone P, Brown RG, Leentjens AF, McDonald WM, Starkstein S, Weintraub D, Poewe W, Rascol O, Sampaio C, Stebbins GT, Goetz CG. 2007. Depression rating scales in Parkinson's disease: critique and recommendations. Mov Disord 22:1077-1092.
Sheline YI, Mintun MA, Barch DM, Wilkins C, Snyder AZ, Moerlein SM. 2004. Decreased hippocampal 5-HT(2A) receptor binding in older depressed patients using [18F]altanserin positron emission tomography. Neuropsychopharmacology 29:2235-2241.
Smith DF, Stork BS, Wegener G, Ashkanian M, Jakobsen S, Bender D, Audrain H, Vase KH, Hansen SB, Videbech P, Rosenberg R. 2009. [11C]Mirtazapine binding in depressed antidepressant nonresponders studied by PET neuroimaging. Psychopharmacology (Berl) 206:133-140.
Smith DF, Stork BS, Wegener G, Jakobsen S, Bender D, Audrain H, Jensen SB, Hansen SB, Rodell A, Rosenberg R. 2007. Receptor occupancy of mirtazapine determined by PET in healthy volunteers. Psychopharmacology (Berl) 195:131-138.
Sobocki P, Jonsson B, Angst J, Rehnberg C. 2006. Cost of depression in Europe. J Ment Health Policy Econ 9:87-98.
Spanagel R, Weiss F. 1999. The dopamine hypothesis of reward: past and current status. Trends Neurosci 22:521-527.
Sullivan GM, Ogden RT, Oquendo MA, Kumar JS, Simpson N, Huang YY, Mann JJ, Parsey RV. 2009. Positron emission tomography quantification of serotonin-1A receptor binding in medication-free bipolar depression. Biol Psychiatry 66:223-230.

Takikawa S, Dhawan V, Chaly T, Robeson W, Dahl R, Zanzi I, Mandel F, Spetsieris P, Eidelberg D. 1994. Input functions for 6-[fluorine-18]fluorodopa quantitation in parkinsonism: comparative studies and clinical correlations. J Nucl Med 35:955-963.

Tanis KQ, Duman RS. 2007. Intracellular signaling pathways pave roads to recovery for mood disorders. Ann Med 39:531-544.

Thase ME. 2009. Atypical depression: useful concept, but it's time to revise the DSM-IV criteria. Neuropsychopharmacology 34:2633-2641.

Theodore WH, Hasler G, Giovacchini G, Kelley K, Reeves-Tyer P, Herscovitch P, Drevets W. 2007. Reduced hippocampal 5HT1A PET receptor binding and depression in temporal lobe epilepsy. Epilepsia 48:1526-1530.

Tosi G, Costantino L, Ruozi B, Forni F, Vandelli MA. 2008. Polymeric nanoparticles for the drug delivery to the central nervous system. Expert Opin Drug Deliv 5:155-174.

Vergoni AV, Tosi G, Tacchi R, Vandelli MA, Bertolini A, Costantino L. 2009. Nanoparticles as drug delivery agents specific for CNS: in vivo biodistribution. Nanomedicine 5:369-377.

Voineskos AN, Wilson AA, Boovariwala A, Sagrati S, Houle S, Rusjan P, Sokolov S, Spencer EP, Ginovart N, Meyer JH. 2007. Serotonin transporter occupancy of high-dose selective serotonin reuptake inhibitors during major depressive disorder measured with [11C]DASB positron emission tomography. Psychopharmacology (Berl) 193:539-545.

Wegener G, Volke V. 2010. Nitric oxide synthase inhibitors as antidepressants. Pharmaceuticals 3:273-299.

Figure legends

Figure 1. Major molecular pathways involved in neuroplasticity and affected by stress, depression, and antidepressant treatment. Some major molecular pathways involved in both short- and long-term neuroplastic changes are shown. Certain intermediates and other details are left out for clarity. Many of these pathways are influenced in opposite ways by stress and depression. For example, both chronic stress in animals and depression in humans have been associated with reductions in the transcription factor CREB, and antidepressants enhance CREB activity in the hippocampus. Abbreviations: NMDA, N-methyl-D-aspartate glutamate receptor; AMPA, amino-3-hydroxy-5-methyl-isoxozole-4-propionic acid glutamate receptor; VGCC, voltage-gated calcium channel;
5-HT, 5-hydroxytryptamine (serotonin); NE, norepinephrine; DA, dopamine; BDNF, brain-derived neurotropic factor; Trk-B, BDNF receptor; AC, adenylyl cyclase; ATP, adenosine triphosphate; cAMP, cyclic adenosine monophosphate; AMP, adenosine monophosphate; PDE, phosphodiesterase, CaMK, calcium-calmodulin-dependent kinase; PKC, protein kinase C; MAPK, mitogen-activated protein kinase; PKA, protein kinase A; Rsk, ribosomal S6 protein kinase; CREB, cAMP response element-binding protein. Reprinted by permission from Macmillan Publishers Ltd: *Neuropsychopharmacology*, Pittinger, C. and Duman, R.S., 33: 88-109, copyright 2008.

Figure 2. The selective 5-HT_{1A} receptor antagonist WAY-100635 which can be labelled on the methyl position to give [*O-methyl*-^{11}C]WAY-100635 or the carbonyl position to give [*carbonyl*-^{11}C]WAY-100635. Labelling positions are indicated with (*).

Figure 1

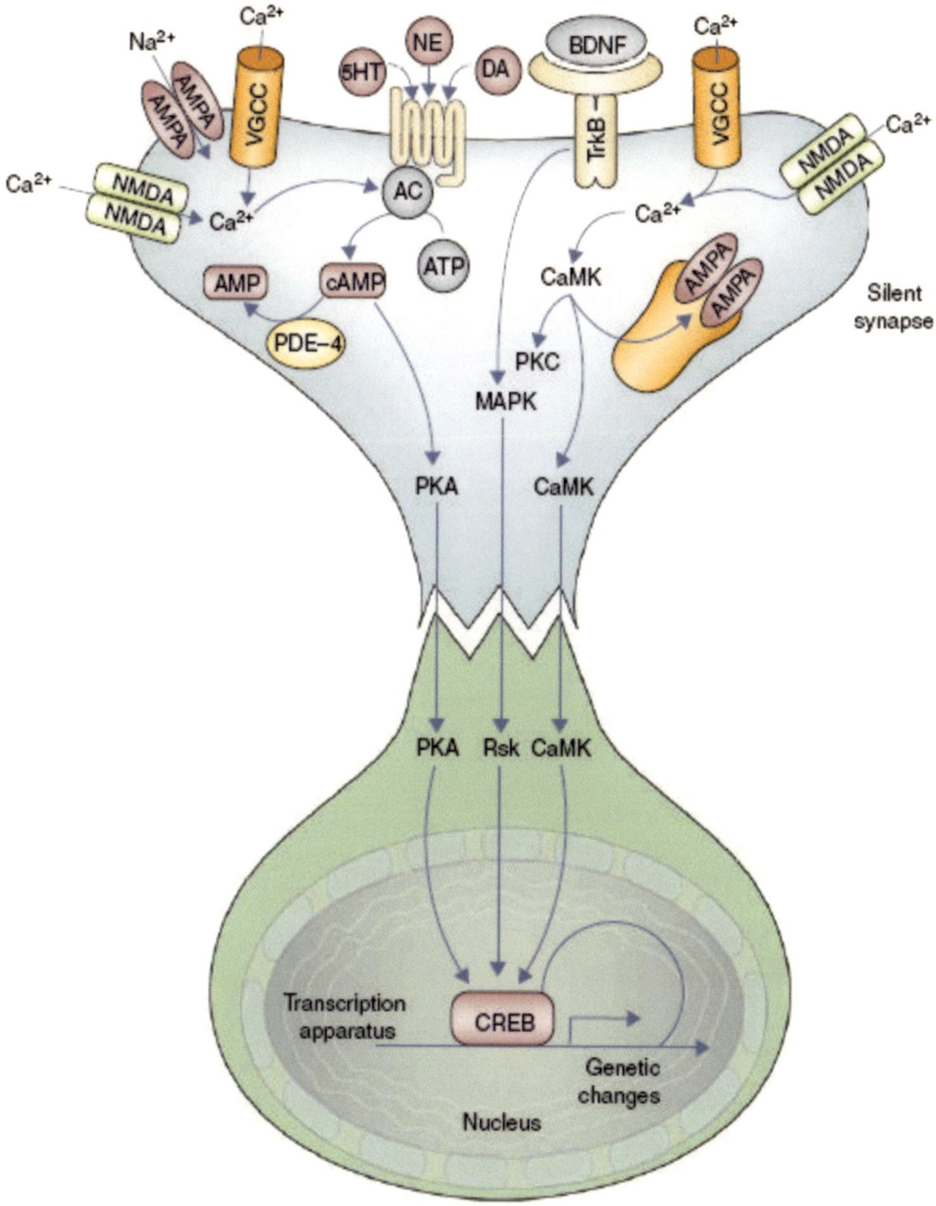

Ca²⁺
Na²⁺
AMPA
AMPA
VGCC
NE
5HT
DA
BDNF
TrkB
Ca²⁺
VGCC
NMDA
NMDA
Ca²⁺
Ca²⁺
NMDA
NMDA
Ca²⁺
AC
Ca²⁺
AMP
cAMP
ATP
CaMK
AMPA
AMPA
Silent synapse
PDE-4
PKC
MAPK
PKA
CaMK
PKA
Rsk
CaMK
Transcription apparatus
CREB
Genetic changes
Nucleus

Figure 2

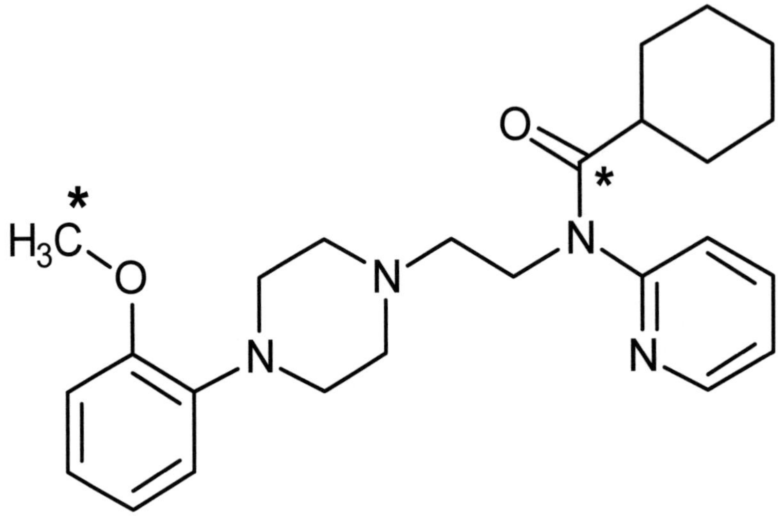

5

Neurobiology of substance-related addiction: findings of neuroimaging

Nina Seiferth and Andreas Heinz
Department of Psychiatry and Psychotherapy
Charité - Universitätsmedizin Berlin
Germany

1. From consumption to addiction: understanding the course of disease

Current research on alcohol and drug dependence gradually showed that the development of addiction has to be understood as a complex interplay of psychological factors and neurobiological adaptation processes induced by consumption-related behavioural changes. Therefore, we review the results of recent neuroimaging research in humans that tried to understand the development of drug addiction in each of its stages. After giving an introduction to the imaging techniques and to the main neuroanatomical and -chemical targets of addiction research, we review changes in the brains' neuronal networks and in relevant neurotransmitter systems related to the processing of substance-related stimuli. We continue by reporting alterations in attention networks and memory formation, which are considered to be relevant for sustaining drug intake. We proceed by outlining imaging results on phenomena which are considered to define addiction itself like craving and withdrawal. Finally, we give an overview on neuroimaging research on relapse risk. We conclude with some comments on possible therapeutical implications of recent imaging results and on future perspectives.

1.1 Methodological approaches

Technical improvement in the neurosciences has provided powerful tools for research on functional brain activity related to addictive behaviour in humans. There are different imaging techniques which are most commonly used during the last decade. Since the neuroscientific methods used also give us information about scientific questions which could not yet be answered, the available imaging methods will shortly be addressed from a methodological point of view.

One way to understand the brains' functional organisation is using the functional Magnetic Resonance Imaging (fMRI) technique. This method allows for indirectly assessing neuronal activity by measuring changes in local blood flow. In detail, it measures the ratio of oxygenated and des-oxygenated blood, the so called blood oxygen level dependent (BOLD) contrast. This allows for an estimation of the underlying neural activity, since it has been shown that changes in blood flow and blood oxygenation are linked to neuronal activity (Kwong et al., 1992; Logothetis, 2002; Ogawa et al., 1990). fMRI is one of the most prominent neuroimaging techniques because of its non-invasiveness, the lack of radiation exposure, the relatively high availability and its good spatial resolution. Disadvantages of the method are the rather poor temporal resolution (e.g. versus EEG), the lack of an absolute baseline of activity and the fact that specific neurotransmitter systems can not be systematically assessed without applying specific agonists/ antagonists.

In contrast to fMRI, the so called Positron Emission Tomography (PET) as well as Single Photon Emission Computed Tomography (SPECT) allow for measurement of an absolute baseline of activation. Furthermore, these imaging methods can quantify neuroreceptor and transporter availabilities, although a potential confound of endogenous neurotransmitter concentration competing for binding of receptors/ transporters with radioligands has to be taken into account (Heinz et al., 2004a; Kumakura et al., 2007; Laruelle 2000).

Clear disadvantages of PET and SPECT measurements are the application of a radioactive contrast agent exposing the subject to gamma radiation, the often rather short half-life period of the commonly used tracers and the rather high expenses required.

An elegant way to link specific brain functions with certain neurotransmitter systems, like linking dopamine with the brain reward system, is to use the combination of both methods: the correlation of neuronal activation measured with fMRI and functions of neurotransmitter system measured with PET or SPECT, e.g. dopamine receptor D_2 availability or dopamine synthesis rate (Kienast et al., 2008).

1.2 Neuroanatomical core structures

Considerable progress has been made during the last two decades in the attempt to identify the basic neuronal mechanisms that underlie addictive behaviour. Animal studies revealed that alcohol- and drug-associated cues activate dopamine and endorphin release in the medial prefrontal cortex and the ventral striatum including the nucleus accumbens, a core area of the brains' reward system (Dayas et al., 2007; Di Chiara, 2002; Shalev et al., 2000). As already mentioned, functional brain activity related to addictive behaviour in humans can be indirectly assessed by measuring changes in cerebral blood flow with PET, SPECT or by measuring the BOLD response with fMRI. These neuroscientific techniques gain insight into the neurobiology of addiction when combined with paradigms, which are designed to study single components of addiction and its development, e.g. so-called "cue-reactivity" paradigms (e.g. Braus et al., 2001; Drummond, 2000; George et al., 2001; Grüsser et al., 2004). As it might be expected, studies reveal differing results regarding the main neuroanatomical regions of interest, depending e.g. on the specific paradigm used and on inter-individual differences in the functional neuroanatomy related to addiction. Nevertheless, there are some core regions in the brain which are repeatedly activated by drug-specific stimuli across studies: 1. The anterior cingulate cortex (ACC) and the adjacent medial prefrontal cortex. This brain region is considered to be involved in processes encoding the motivational value of a stimulus. Therefore, it is also of importance for attention and memory processes (Grüsser et al., 2004; Heinz et al., 2004b; Myrick et al., 2004; Tapert et al., 2004). 2. The orbitofrontal cortex (OFC). This brain area has been related to the evaluation of the reward value of processed stimuli (Myrick et al., 2004; Wrase et al., 2002). 3. The amygdala, mainly the basolateral part. The amygdala is known to represent the emotional salience of stimuli and it is involved in unconditioned and conditioned approach and avoidance behaviour (Schneider et al., 2001). 4. The ventral striatum including the nucleus accumbens. These brain regions are considered to code the motivational aspects of salient stimuli and to link with motor reactions (Wrase et al., 2007; Braus et al., 2001; Wrase et al., 2002). 5. The dorsal striatum. It has been implicated in habit formation and the consolidation of stimulus-reaction-patterns (Grüsser et al., 2004; Modell & Mountz, 1995). 6. The dorsolateral prefrontal cortex (DLPFC). It contributes to the executive control of behaviour and might therefore be relevant for resisting craving for the substance of abuse (George et al., 2001) and to guide behavioural adaptation and learning (Park et al., 2010).

1.3 Relevant neurotransmitter systems

Beside the main neuroanatomical correlates of the development of alcohol and drug addiction, modern imaging methods like PET provide a powerful tool for the systematic examination of the underlying neurotransmitter systems and their changes. The first relevant neurotransmitter to mention in the context of the development of addiction is dopamine. All drugs of abuse are known to release dopamine, which reinforces drug-taking behaviour (Di Chiara & Bassareo, 2007) and chronically induces counter-adaptive processes such as receptor down-regulation (Koob, 2003). To give an example, PET studies in detoxified alcoholic showed a reduction of availability and sensitivity of central dopamine D_2-receptors, which can serve as an example of a neuroadaptive process after chronic alcohol consumption, which was further associated with the subsequent relapse risk (Heinz et al., 1996; Volkow et al., 1996).

A different mechanism is implicated by sensitisation: Neuroadaptation in terms of long-term sensitisation towards the effects of drugs and drug-associated stimuli can be caused by structural changes in striatal GABAergic neurons, which are innervated by dopaminergic neurons and play a major role in the signal transfer towards the thalamus and the cortex (Robinson & Kolb, 1997). Drugs like alcohol also appear to directly stimulate GABA receptors and inhibits the function of glutamatergic NMDA-receptors (Kalivas & Volkow, 2005; Krystal et al., 2006).

The cannabinoid and opioidergic system are other neurotransmitter systems, which are involved in the development and maintenance of drug abuse. High concentrations of CB1-receptors are found in the prefrontal cortex, the ventral tegmental area, the amygdala, the hippocampus, and the ventral striatum including the nucleus accumbens, i.e. structures which are known to be of high relevance for addiction development. Further, CB1-receptors modulate the release of dopamine, GABA and glutamate and elicit long-term changes in synaptic neurotransmission, like long-term potentiation or depression (De Vries & Schoffelmeer, 2005), which may play a role in addiction-specific neuroadaptations.

2. Learning to maintain consumption

Brain-imaging studies have increasingly focused on the early phase of disease, i.e. researchers are more and more interested in identifying addiction-specific risk factors as well as in describing the initial behavioural processes and the resulting neuronal changes. Therefore, current imaging studies try to identify the neuronal correlates of learning processes including classical Pavlovian and instrumental conditioning involved in disease development as well as in the risk of relapse. On the one hand, the goal of such studies is to provide insight into the neurobiology of drug addiction and therefore to improve understanding of the brain. On the other hand, researches intend to provide new options for specific behavioural interventions or psychopharmacological modification of alcohol craving and the risk of relapse.

2.1 Contextual cues

One important factor in the development of addiction is the occurrence of conditioned reactions elicited by conditioned cues, i.e. stimuli that have previously been associated with alcohol or drug consumption. For example, if an originally neutral stimulus (UCS), like a drinking glass, has been regularly associated with the consumption of a substance of abuse, like wine or other alcoholic beverages, the stimulus will also be associated with the positively experienced effects of alcohol as an unconditioned response (UCR) and turns into a conditioned stimulus (CS). As a consequence, this stimulus can itself provoke consumption or associated behavior as a conditioned response (CR; see Figure 1).

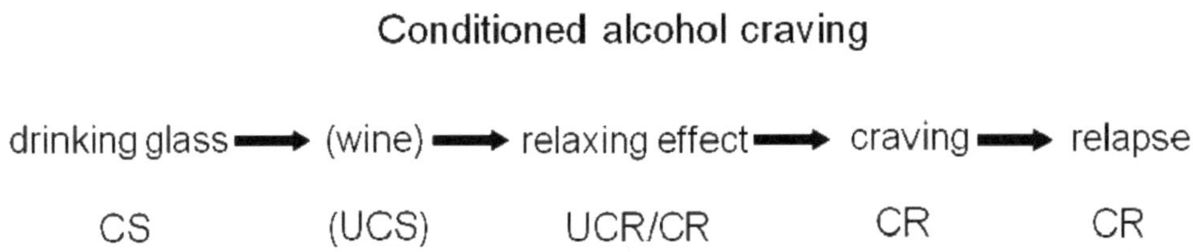

Fig. 1. Model of conditioned alcohol consumption: a previously unconditioned stimulus (UCS; e.g. wine glass) is regularly associated with alcohol consumption. Thus, it becomes associated with the alcohol effect as an unconditioned response (UCR) and changes to a conditioned stimulus (CS). The CS itself is then able to elicit alcohol craving and even relapse as a conditioned response (CR).

In opiate addiction, studies in animals and humans demonstrated that heroin-associated environmental cues triggered conditioned reactions that counteract the expected drug effect (Wikler, 1948; Siegel et al., 1975, 1982). Rodents which received opiate always in the same cage showed a rather high tolerance to the opiate effects until they received the same dose in a different cage. In the latter case, the conditioned counter-adaptive response did not occur and the animals died of an overdose of opiate. On the other hand, the animals showed symptoms of opiate withdrawal if they did not receive the expected opiate dose after being exposed to the contextual cue, i.e. the habitual cage. Likewise in humans, cues characterizing situations of alcohol or drug intake and their associated effects may act as conditioned stimuli that trigger counter-adaptive alterations in neurotransmission. Such changes may manifest as subjectively aversive withdrawal symptoms and lead to repeated drug intake, i.e. trigger relapse (Verheul et al., 1999).

2.2 Reward-associated changes in salience

If a person is repeatedly exposed to a drug or alcohol intake, different neuroadaptive changes are considered to happen. One important aspect is that our brains' attentional network is highly effective in learning to react to contextual or internal stimuli which are of high relevance, i.e. of high salience. Robinson and Berridge (1993) suggested that phasic dopamine release facilitates the allocation of attention towards salient, reward-indicating stimuli, which can motivate the individual to show a particular behaviour to achieve the reward. With that assumption they referred to a fundamental work by Schultz and colleagues, who had observed that the occurrence of unexpected rewarding stimuli elicits a burst of spikes in dopaminergic neurons (Schultz et al., 1997). In contrast, if its appearance is signaled by a conditioned cue, the discharge of the dopaminergic neurons occurs already with the perception of the conditioned cue, and the rewarding stimulus itself does no longer elicit a discharge of dopamine. These results were remarkable, as Schultz and coworkers also showed that the absence of an expected reward after the occurrence of a conditioned cue leads to a transient cessation of dopamine neuron firing directly after the moment when the expected reward does not arrive (see Figure 2). Thus, the dopaminergic system indicates unexpected reward as well as the non-appearance of expected reinforcers, i.e. it serves as an error-detection signal and therefore contributes to learning, goal directed behaviour as well as behavioural flexibility. Furthermore, the dopamine signal reflects the magnitude of the anticipated reward (Tobler et al., 2005). Thus, the nucleus accumbens may act as a "sensory motor gateway" controlling the effects of salient contextual stimuli on prefrontal brain areas and limbic regions which regulate attention as well as motor behaviour.

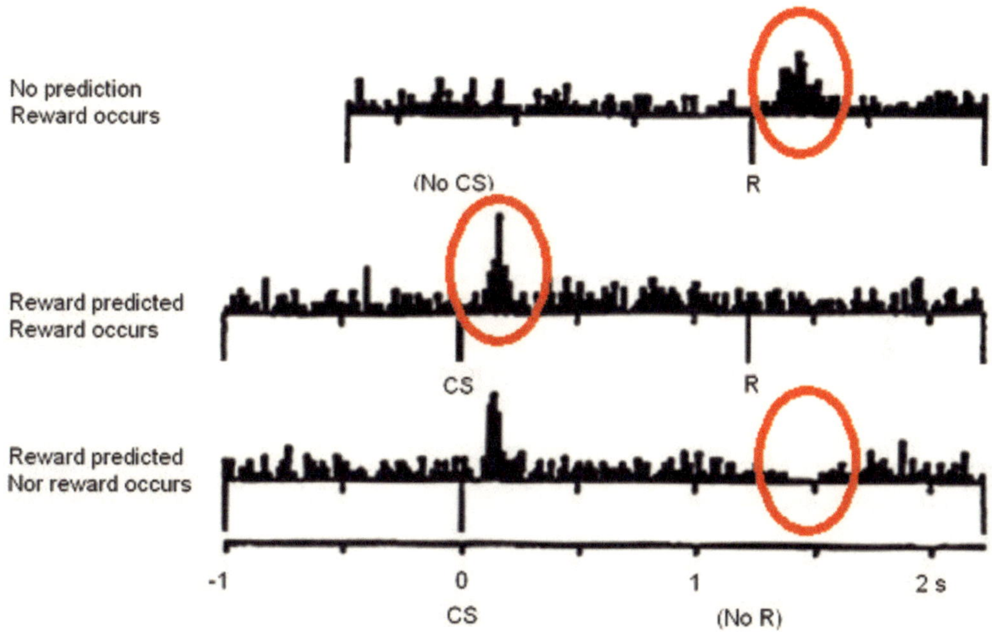

Fig. 2. Reward-associated phasic dopamine release (Schulz et al., 1997). *Top*: Unexpected and unpredicted reward (banana pellets for rhesus monkeys) is reflected in a short term increase in dopamine firing. *Middle*: After having learned that a light (conditioned stimulus, CS) regularly predicts a reward (R), the appearance of the CS generates a short-term increase in phasic dopamine firing rate. The reward itself is now completely predicted by the CS and does not elicit dopamine firing. *Bottom*: If a CS is not followed by the expected reward, an error in reward prediction occurs (unexpected lack of reward), which is reflected in a phasic decrease in dopamine firing.

In humans, few studies directly examined the correlation between cue-induced brain activation and dopamine dysfunction or changes in other neurotransmitter systems such as glutamate or GABA. Studies showed that in detoxified alcohol-dependent patients, the extent of alcohol craving was correlated with both a low dopamine synthesis capacity measured with F-DOPA PET and with a reduced availability of dopamine D_2-receptors in the ventral striatum (Heinz et al., 2005b; Heinz et al., 2004b). This reduction was correlated with an increased activation of the anterior cingulate and adjacent medial prefrontal cortex measured with fMRI during the processing of alcohol-related versus neutral control stimuli (Heinz et al., 2004b). Interestingly, these brain areas have been associated with attention attribution to salient stimuli (Fuster et al., 1997). It seems surprising that alcohol-associated stimuli should provoke an increase in brain activation in attention network although all other contextual cues, in this case a loud and noisy MRI scanner, indicate that there is no chance for obtaining alcohol. One possible explanation is based on the work of Schultz and colleagues (1997) who demonstrated that phasic alterations in dopamine release are not only required to learn new stimulus-reward associations but also that they may be necessary to "unlearn" established associations. In this phase of dependence, low dopamine synthesis, reduced stimulus-induced dopamine release and diminished D_2-receptor availability in the ventral striatum (Heinz et al., 2005b; Heinz et al., 2004b; Martinez et al., 2005) may interfere with dopamine-dependent processing of errors in reward expectation (Heinz et al., 2004b). Moving attention away from drug-associated conditioned stimuli and diminishing the attributed salience of such cues might be of specific difficulty for drug-dependent patients. Signaling of the potential availability of alcohol or the drug of abuse has been well learned, for example via glutamate-dependent long-term potentiation within the ventral hippocampus-ventral striatal pathway which has been associated with perseverative behaviour (Goto & Grace, 2005). In accordance with this hypothesis, a linear correlation between increased alcohol cue-induced activation of the medial prefrontal cortex and the reduction of dopamine D_2-receptor availability in the ventral striatum was found in detoxified alcoholics, further underlining that the degree of dopamine dysfunction may contribute to excessive salience attribution to alcohol-associated cues (Heinz et al., 2004b). Also in clinical experience, many detoxified alcohol-dependent patients report difficulty to remain abstinent when being confronted with scenes which still are of high salience for drug intake, i.e. typical drinking situations like someone sitting lonely on the sofa and watching TV ads for an alcoholic beverage.

Moving one step further, first studies indicate why the process of re-learning non-addictive behaviour seems so difficult to initiate: due to the described changes within the phasic characteristics of dopaminergic neurotransmission, alcohol-dependent patients may have problems in attributing salience to newly learned conditioned stimuli indicating the availability of non-drug reward. Wrase and colleagues (2007) observed a reduction in functional activation in the ventral striatum when being confronted with non-drug-associated, reward-indicating cues in alcoholics. Moreover, the reduced activation was correlated with the severity of alcohol craving and could not be explained by performance differences or mood. Reduced activation of the striatum to new, reward-indicating stimuli might therefore reflect the patients' diminished motivation to experience new and potentially rewarding situations. Interestingly, the same patients showed an increased activity of the ventral striatum when being confronted with alcohol-associated stimuli, which was also correlated with the severity of alcohol craving. Such a finding is in line with the prominent hypothesis that substances of abuse "hijack" the reward system and stabilize a dysfunctional state, i.e. when the ventrial striatum primarily responds to drug-associated stimuli while the adequate processing of conventional, primary reinforcing stimuli such as food or sex is impeded (Volkow et al., 2004). Further research is needed to elucidate neuronal processing of natural reinforcers in addiction as well as (reversal) learning in general. For clinical practice, these findings also improve our understanding why it can be difficult to motivate detoxified alcoholics to replace alcohol by other reinforcers such as social interactions or new activities: their brains' response to alternative reward-indicating stimuli tends to be reduced in relevant brain regions. This may make it very difficult to - literally spoken - concentrate oneself on other aspects of the world than cues associated with the drug of abuse.

2.3 Modification in emotional response

One milestone of neurobiological research on alcohol and drug addiction is the observation that alcohol and all other drugs of abuse induce dopamine release in the ventral striatum, including the nucleus accumbens, and thus reinforce drug intake (Wise, 1988). Although a drug thus "reinforces" a specific behaviour, this does not necessarily imply that the drug effect is also subjectively pleasant. In a commonly known work by Robinson and Berridge (1993) the authors suggested to distinguish between the hedonic, i.e. pleasant, drug effects ("liking") and the feeling of craving for such a positive effect ("wanting"). Further, they attributed these effects to different neurotransmitter systems. They suggested that neurobiological effects associated with "liking" the drug are mediated by opioidergic neurotransmission in the ventral striatum, including the nucleus accumbens. This assumption was based on the observation that hedonic effects during consumption of a drug are caused by endorphin release in these brain areas - like during the consumption of primarily reinforcing stimuli such as food (Berridge & Robinson, 1998). Based on the work of Schultz and colleagues (1997), Berridge and Robinson further suggested that the neurobiological correlate of "wanting" is (phasic) dopamine release in the ventral striatum. Following imaging studies intended to evaluate these aspects of the reward system - on a neurobiological as well as on a behavioural level by additionally using questionnaires for drug craving as a proxy for "wanting" beside scales measuring pleasure as a proxy for "liking". Indeed, studies suggested that acute drug craving is associated with dopamine dysfunction in the ventral striatum, i.e. reduced dopamine synthesis and D_2-receptor availability (Heinz et al., 2005b), while increased μ-opiate receptors in the ventral striatum correlated with other aspects of chronic alcohol intake and alcohol urges (Heinz et al., 2005a).

2.4 Memory formation

Striatal dopamine release is regulated by the hippocampus, which is well known to play a major role in memory formation (Lisman & Grace, 2005). In rats that had formerly consumed cocaine, the stimulation of glutamatergic neurons in the hippocampus resulted in dopamine release in the ventral striatum and led to renewed drug intake (Vorel et al., 2001). Experimental stimulation of the hippocampus may reflect real-life situations in which contextual, drug-associated cues activate the hippocampus and thus trigger memories associated with previous drug use (see Figure 3). In such situations, the activation of the

described hippocampus-VTA circuit will activate dopamine neurons in the VTA, which elicit dopamine release in the ventral striatum, thus facilitating new drug intake (Floresco et al., 2001). Indeed it has been shown that both cocaine and amphetamine sensitization (Goto & Grace, 2005; Lodge & Grace, 2008) increases hippocampal input in the nucleus accumbens, finally resulting in aggravated responses of the dopaminergic system.
Hyman (2005) argued that addiction somehow represents neuroadaptive processes in learning and memory that - under normal circumstances - serve to shape survival behaviour, i.e. behaviour related to the pursuit of rewards and the cues that predict them. Beside the possibility of synapse elimination and remodelling, the best known mechanisms of synaptic plasticity in learning and memory are such phenomena that change the strength or "weight" of existing connections, so called long-term potentiation and long-term depression. Although most of relevant research is based on animal models, long-term potentiation and depression have become important candidate mechanisms for the drug-induced alterations of neural circuits that are posited to occur with addiction in humans. There is evidence that both mechanisms occur in the nucleus accumbens and other targets of mesolimbic dopamine neurons as a consequence of drug administration, and growing literature suggests that they may play an important role in the development of addiction. The underlying molecular mechanisms include regulation of the phosphorylation state of key proteins, alterations in the availability of glutamate receptors at the synapse and regulation of gene expression (for review see e.g. Hyman & Malenka, 2001; Kauer et al., 2004; Thomas & Malenka, 2003).

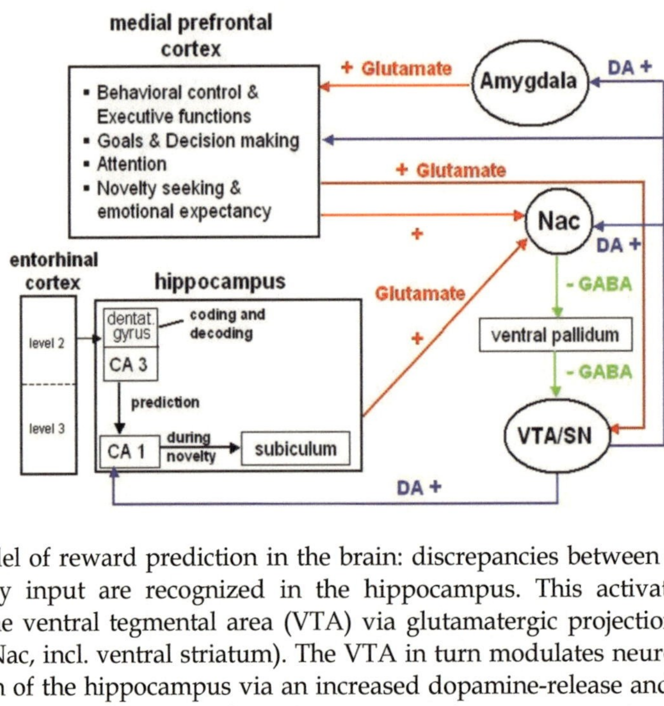

Fig. 3. A model of reward prediction in the brain: discrepancies between the expected and actual sensory input are recognized in the hippocampus. This activates dopaminergic neurons in the ventral tegmental area (VTA) via glutamatergic projections to the nucleus accumbens (Nac, incl. ventral striatum). The VTA in turn modulates neuronal transmission in CA1 region of the hippocampus via an increased dopamine-release and thus contributes to memory modification. The prefrontal cortex contributes to executive control functions and modulates the firing rate of dopaminergic neurons that project from the VTA region to the Nac and the amygdala (modified from Lisman & Grace, 2005).

3. Developing addiction

3.1 Criteria of addiction

Alcohol dependence and other drug addictions are characterized by criteria such as tolerance development, withdrawal symptoms, drug craving and reduced control of drug intake (American Psychiatric Association, 2000; World Health Organization, 2007). For the development of tolerance, it has been suggested that this phenomenon is based on a process of neuroadaptation in the brain to chronically increased alcohol or drug consumption. Continued drug intake leads to an anticipatory compensation of the drugs' effects by the brain, which results in a new homeostatic balance. This adapted state of equilibrium is disturbed when drug or alcohol intake is suddenly interrupted, as it is the case during detoxification. This can result in clinically manifest withdrawal symptoms, which are opposed to the drugs primary physiological and psychological effects (Koob, 2003). For instance, alcohols' sedative effects are mediated by inhibition of glutamatergic and stimulation of GABAergic neurotransmission (Tsai et al., 1995; Krystal et al., 2006). Insufficient GABAergic inhibition and increased glutamatergic excitation may result in highly aversive withdrawal symptoms and in epileptic seizures (Tsai et al., 1995; Krystal et al., 2006). Many imaging studies have focused on the neurobiological correlates of the defining characteristics of addiction in order to gain insight into the essence of the disease.

3.2 Craving

Within cue-reactivity paradigms, the reported correlations between subjectively reported craving and the actual consumptive behaviour are often low. This may in parts be explained by the different levels the reaction can emerge on (subjective, motor, physiological) and which are associated with different degrees of consciousness. Tiffany (1990) described a cognitive model in which conscious craving only occurs if an automatic process of drug intake is interrupted, which may be triggered by conditioned stimuli and motivate for drug intake even in the absence of conscious drug urges.

Unfortunately, imaging results regarding cue-induced activity in the brain and subjective craving for alcohol or other drugs are not very consistent. Myrick and colleagues (2004) reported an association between the severity of craving and functional brain activation in the ventral striatum, orbitofrontal cortex and anterior cingulate cortex, while others described such a relationship for the dorsal striatum (Modell & Mountz, 1995) or the subcallosal gyrus (Tapert et al., 2004). Further studies were not able to identify any significant correlation between alcohol craving and cue-induced brain activation (Grüsser et al., 2004; Heinz et al., 2004b). Trying to understand these diverging findings, one has to take into account that all studies used different stimuli for craving induction: alcohol-related words (Tapert et al., 2004), alcohol-related pictures with (Myrick et al., 2004) or without (Grüsser et al., 2004) a sip of alcohol ("priming dose"). Furthermore, time point of examination differed from patients being not detoxified (Myrick et al., 2004) to detoxified patients in an inpatient treatment program (Braus et al., 2001; Grüsser et al., 2004; Heinz et al., 2004b; Heinz et al., 2007; Wrase et al., 2002; Wrase et al., 2007).

3.3 Habit formation

For the development of addiction, specifically for reduced control of drug intake, it is of high relevance (Robbins & Everitt, 2002) to understand the behavioural transfer from conscious consumption to a more automated behaviour, i.e. forming a habit (Tiffany, 1990). It has been suggested that the dorsal striatum is crucial for habit learning, i.e. for the learning of automated responses, and may thus contribute to the compulsive character of dependent behaviour.

The importance of habitual drug intake for the development of addiction appears to be reflected in anatomical changes associated with cue-induced activation: whilst reward-driven striatal reactivity is known to predominantly involve the ventral striatum, cue-induced conscious craving in addicted subjects may preferentially elicit dopamine release in more dorsal striatal structures (Volkow et al., 2006; Wong et al., 2006). Such a transition from a predominantly ventral response to the dorsal striatum might reflect a change from a reward-driven activity of the ventral striatum to a more automated stimulus-response habit formation depending on dorsal striatal activity (Berke & Hyman, 2000). The rewarding effect of e.g. ventral striatal dopamine release may play a subordinate role in such automated processes, what is in line with the clinical impression and reports of patients. In accordance, Robbins and Everitt (2002) proposed that the initially reinforcing effect of drugs of abuse is based on the activation of the ventral striatum, while the transfer into habitual drug-seeking is associated with activation of more dorsal striatal regions. Studies with PET could also support that assumption, since among addicted subjects, drug cues preferentially lead to dopamine release in the dorsal striatum and putamen (Volkow et al., 2006; Wong et al., 2006). In line with the research, many patients also describe their relapse in terms of automated actions and do not remember to have experienced craving before relapse as in earlier stages of disease development (Tiffany, 1990).

3.4 Neurochemical adaptation underlying the development of addiction

Different neurotransmitter systems are involved in the processing of rewarding stimuli in general and of addiction-related phenomena in particular (see 1.3. for an overview). For a long time, neurobiological research on addiction mainly focussed on dopamine dysfunctions but in the recent past it has broaden its view on other neurotransmitter systems.

Brain imaging studies with PET clearly showed a reduced availability and sensitivity of central dopamine D_2-receptors in alcohol-dependent patients - potentially reflecting a compensatory down-regulation after chronic alcohol intake, which was associated with the subsequent relapse risk (Heinz et al., 1996; Volkow et al., 1996). Following PET studies (F-DOPA PET) revealed that alcohol craving was specifically correlated with a low dopamine synthesis capacity and with reduced dopamine D_2-receptor availability in the ventral striatum including the nucleus accumbens (Heinz et al., 2004b; Heinz et al., 2005b). Animal experiments also showed that extracellular dopamine concentrations decreased rapidly during detoxification (Rossetti et al., 1992). Thus, dopamine dysfunction may further be augmented by reduced intra-synaptic dopamine release during early abstinence. Another PET study (Martinez et al., 2005) showed that dopamine release in detoxified alcoholics was significantly reduced following amphetamine administration. Thus, overall dopaminergic neurotransmission in the ventral striatum of alcohol-dependent patients was reduced after detoxification. Unlike suggested by Robinson and Berridge (1993), it thus might seem unlikely that the appearance of a drug-associated cue can cause a significant dopamine release triggering craving or relapse. Indeed, animal studies demonstrated that alcohol and drug-associated stimuli can lead to relapse even if no dopamine is released in the ventral striatum (Shalev et al., 2002). Nevertheless, a down-regulation rather than a sensitisation of the dopamine system appears to play a role in relapse behaviour: In humans, dopamine dysfunction was correlated with the severity of alcohol craving and with increased processing of alcohol-associated cues in the anterior cingulate and medial prefrontal cortex (Heinz et al., 2004b), brain areas in which an increased reaction on alcohol cues has been associated with an increased relapse risk (Grüsser et al., 2004).

Structural changes in striatal GABAergic neurons have also been considered to account for phenomena of long-term sensitisation towards the effects of drugs and drug-associated stimuli. Striatal GABAergic neurons are innervated by dopaminergic neurons and play a major role in the signal transfer towards the thalamus and the cortex (Robinson and Kolb, 1997). E.g., alcohol consumption stimulates GABA receptors and inhibits the function of glutamatergic NMDA-receptors (Kalivas & Volkow, 2005; Krystal et al., 2006). The alcohol-induced inhibition of the glutamatergic signal transduction results in up-regulation of NMDA receptors (Schumann et al., 2005; Tsai et al., 1995). As a consequence, the loss of this inhibition of NMDA receptor function via alcohol during early abstinence was related to hyperexcitation and withdrawal symptoms (Spanagel, 2003). Repeated withdrawal in turn elicits an increase in glutamate release (Kalivas et al., 2005). Therefore, it has been suggested that glutamatergic neurotransmission in a brain network spanning the prefrontal cortex, the amygdala, the hippocampus, the nucleus accumbens and the ventral tegmental area plays a major role in triggering relapse (Kalivas et al., 2005). Pharmacological treatment strategies pick up such findings, e.g. acamprosate, a drug used to reduce relapse risk in alcohol-dependent patients, diminishes alcohol craving via modulation of NMDA-receptors (Mann et al., 2004; Spanagel, 2003).

As already noted, the cannabinoid and opioidergic system also play a role in the development and maintenance of addictive behaviour. High concentration of CB1-receptors have been described in relevant brain regions, in detail in the prefrontal cortex, the amygdala, the ventral tegmental area, the hippocampus, the nucleus accumbens and the ventral striatum. In animal models of excessive nicotine and methamphetamine abuse, blockade of CB1-receptors reduced drug intake during relapse (De Vries & Schoffelmeer, 2005). Therefore, CB1-receptors are thought to modulate the activity of other neurotransmitters (dopamine, GABA and glutamate) and elicit long-term changes in synaptic transmission, in detail long-term potentiation or depression. Anyhow, further research is needed here to elicit the complex interplay of these neurotransmitter systems.

Within the opioidergic system, animal studies showed that blockade of μ-opiate receptors with naltrexone reduced dopamine release in the ventral striatum as well as alcohol consumption (Gonzales & Weiss, 1998). In humans, it has been shown that alcohol-dependent patients display an increase of μ-opiate receptors in the ventral striatum, which was further significantly correlated with the amount of craving (Heinz et al., 2005a). In line with that, application of the opiate antagonist naltrexone in humans can reduce alcohol craving and the subjective "liking" of the drug associated with its intake (O'Brien, 2005) and might reduce the risk of relapse in some patients (e.g. Srisurapanont & Jarusuraisin, 2005).

4. Risk of relapse

Detoxification itself does little to prevent subsequent relapse in alcoholics. Up to 85% of all patients relapse in the placebo control groups of treatment studies, even if treated as inpatients until complete remission of physical withdrawal symptoms (Boothby & Doering, 2005). It has been suggested that exposure to stress and to priming doses of alcohol can induce a relapse (Adinoff, 2004; Breese et al., 2005; Cooney, 1997). Another relevant mechanism that contributes to the risk of relapse is the exposure to stimuli that have regularly been associated with alcohol intake (contextual cues). Such stimuli have become conditioned cues that can elicit conditioned responses such as alcohol or drug craving and consumption behaviour (Adinoff, 2004; Berridge & Robinson, 1998; Di Chiara & Bassareo, 2007; Everitt & Robbins 2005). In such situations, patients may experience craving for alcohol or the specific drug, which is based on the natural tendency to avoid unpleasant experiences, e.g. a conditioned withdrawal response to the presentation of drug cues in the absence of drug intake. Indeed, about one third of all alcoholics in a clinical setting described that their relapse was preceded by a sudden manifestation of withdrawal. It often occurred long after acute detoxification and was often triggered by "typical" drinking situations (Heinz et al., 2003).

Although some imaging studies investigated the association between brain activation elicited by alcohol-associated stimuli and alcohol craving (see also 3.2), only few studies assessed to what extent cue-induced brain activation can predict the prospective relapse risk and therefore the clinical relevance of such imaging studies. Braus and colleagues (2001) reported that alcohol cues elicited increased activation of the ventral striatum and visual association cortices in detoxified alcoholics, and that patients who had experienced multiple relapses in the past showed a stronger cue-induced activity in the ventral striatum than patients who successfully abstained from alcohol for longer periods of time. This result was confirmed by Grüsser and colleagues (2004), who compared subsequently relapsing with abstaining patients. The latter group showed less brain activation elicited by visual alcohol-associated stimuli in the anterior cingulate cortex, the adjacent ventral and medial prefrontal cortex and central parts of the striatum. As the striatum, mainly the dorsal part, has been suggested to be crucial for habit learning, this result might reflect differences in the habitual character of addictive behaviour between abstaining and relapsing patients, even in the absence of conscious drug urges ("craving"). These observations are in the line with studies in animals, in which cue-induced relapse after cocaine consumption was prevented by blockade of dopamine and AMPA glutamate receptors in the dorsal striatum (Vanderschuren et al., 2005). Thus, when talking about relapse risk, it seems to be of importance to distinguish between the neuronal correlates of habitual drug intake (i.e. without conscious craving) and drug-intake following the subjective feeling of craving.

Unfortunately, the empirical basis for coherence between craving for the substance of abuse and risk of relapse is not fully satisfying. Although animal models strongly support the hypothesis that conditioned drug reactions are involved in the development and maintenance of addictive behaviour as well as relapse (Di Chiara, 2002; Robbins &Everitt, 2002; Robinson & Berridge, 1993), studies in humans are rather heterogeneous. While some studies did not find a positive correlation between subjective i.e. conscious craving and relapse (Drummond & Glautier, 1994; Grüsser et al., 2004; Junghanns et al., 2005; Kiefer et al., 2005; Litt et al., 2000; Rohsenow et al., 1994), others did show significant correlations (Bottlender & Soyka, 2004; Cooney et al., 1997; Heinz et al., 2005b; Ludwig & Wikler, 1974; Monti et al., 1990). In contrast, changes in physiological parameters, including neuronal activation measured with functional imaging, seem to be more closely connected to relapse (Abrams et al., 1988; Braus et al., 2001; Drummond & Glautier, 1994; Grüsser et al., 2004;

Rohsenow et al., 1994). Linking relapse risk with physiological responses may therefore be a more promising approach, and was used in several studies.
To measure the effects of reactions to non-alcoholic, affectively positive and negative stimuli on the relapse risk, Heinz and colleagues (2007) briefly presented affective pictures to alcoholics versus control subjects while conducting fMRI measurements. The affectively positive pictures elicited increased brain activation in alcoholics in ventral striatum, which was negatively correlated with the subsequent relapse risk and may represent a protective factor against relapse.
Dysfunctions of brain areas associated with executive control of behaviour (see also Figure 3) may also contribute to relapse risk. Indeed, in methamphetamine-dependent patients, the subsequent relapse risk was predicted by activation patterns elicited during a two-choice decision-making task in the insula, posterior cingulate and temporal cortex (Paulus et al., 2005). Similarly, Brewer and colleagues (2008) reported in cocaine dependent patients undergoing a stroop task an increased activation in regions relevant for cognitive control, including the anterior cingulate cortex, dorsolateral prefrontal cortex, as well as in the parietal lobule, insula and striatum. Longer duration of self-reported abstinence correlated with the strength of the activation of the ventromedial prefrontal cortex, left posterior cingulate cortex, and right striatum, percent drug-free urine screenings correlated with striatal activation, and treatment retention correlated with diminished activation of dorsolateral prefrontal cortex. Despite these promising examples, to date only few imaging studied followed the approach to predict relapse risk from the activity of brain areas associated with executive control of behaviour.

5. Clinical implications

Previous research in addiction suggests different therapeutic consequences. First of all, functional imaging studies help to understand the course of addiction development from its beginning up to its manifest state. Further, it can help to identify patients who are particularly at risk to relapse. As the described imaging techniques such as fMRI and PET are rather expensive, the transmission of these results on the application of less complicated techniques, which assess physiological responses to drug-associated cues, might be useful, e.g. the affect-modulated startle response (Heinz et al., 2003). Physiological markers that reflect an appetitive response towards drug cues - such as the startle response - are also important to identify unconscious aspects of craving behaviour, because many patients deny subjective craving when being exposed to a drug-associated cue but show strong appetitive reactions when assessed with the startle response (Heinz et al., 2003).
Patients suffering from strong cue-reactivity and a high risk of relapse may specifically profit from specific psychotherapeutic treatments such as cue exposure. Although, cue exposure has repeatedly been investigated in evaluative studies on the average, this treatment approach does not seem to result in significantly better outcome than standard therapy with cognitive-behavioural therapy and supportive interventions (Kavanagh et al., 2004; Löber et al., 2006). However, cue exposure may work best among patients with strong neuronal responses to alcohol cues, i.e. the identification of a subgroup of such patients may help to provide successful treatment strategies.
Brain imaging is also used to assess the effects of additive pharmacotherapy on cue-induced neuronal activation patterns during abstinence (e.g. Hermann et al., 2006). Myrick and

colleagues (2008) were able to show that cue-induced activation of limbic brain areas is reduced by naltrexone and by the combination of naltrexone and ondansetron in detoxified alcoholics. Since alterations in the response to affective cues have been suggested to predict relapse (Heinz et al., 2007) these results may help to identify new pharmacological and psychological treatment strategies, such as the modulation of the central stress response (e.g. George et al., 2008).

6. References

Abrams, D.B.; Monti, P.M.; Carey, K.B.; Pinto, R.P. & Jacobus, S.I. (1988). Reactivity to smoking cues and relapse - two studies of discriminant validity. *Behaviour Research and Therapy,* 26, 3, 225–233, 0005-7967

Adinoff, B. (2004). Neurobiologic processes in drug reward and addiction. *Harvard Review of Psychiatry,* 12, 305–320, 1067-3229

American Psychiatric Association (2000). *Diagnostic and Statistical Manual of Mental Disorders,* 4th ed., text revision, Washington DC, American Psychiatric Press.

Berke, J.D. & Hyman, S.E. (2000). Addiction, dopamine, and the molecular mechanisms of memory. *Neuron,* 25, 3, 515-532, 0896-6273

Berridge, K.C. & Robinson, T.E. (1998). What is the role of dopamine in reward: hedonic impact, reward learning, or incentive salience? *Brain Research Reviews,* 28, 3, 309–369, 0165-0173

Boothby, L.A. & Doering, P.L. (2005). A camprosate for the treatment of alcohol dependence. *Clinical Therapeutics,* 27, 6, 695–714, 0149-2918

Bottlender, M. & Soyka, M. (2004). Impact of craving on alcohol relapse during, and 12 months following, outpatient treatment. *Alcohol and Alcoholism,* 39, 4, 357–361, 0735-0414

Braus, D.F.; Wrase, J.; Grüsser, S.; Hermann, D.; Ruf, M.; Flor, H.; Mann, K. & Heinz, A. (2001). Alcohol-associated stimuli activate the ventral striatum in abstinent alcoholics. *Journal of Neural Transmission,* 108, 7, 887–894, 0300-9564

Breese, G.R.; Chu, K.; Dayas, C.V.; Funk, D.; Knapp, D.J.; Koob, G.F.; Lê, D.A.; O'Dell, L.E.; Overstreet, D.H.; Roberts, A.J.; Sinha, R.; Valdez, G.R. & Weiss, F. (2005). Stress enhancement of craving during sobriety: a risk for relapse. *Alcoholism: Clinical and Experimental Research,* 29, 2, 185–195, 0145-6008

Brewer, J.A.; Worhunsky, P.D.; Carroll, K.M.; Rounsaville, B.J. & Potenza, M.N. (2008). Pre-Treatment Brain Activation During Stroop Task is Associated with Outcomes in Cocaine Dependent Patients. *Biological Psychiatry,* 64, 11, 998–1004, 0006-3223

Cooney, N.L.; Litt, M.D.; Morse, P.A.; Bauer, L.O. & Gaupp, L. (1997). Alcohol cue reactivity, negative-mood reactivity, and relapse in treated alcoholic men. *Journal of Abnormal Psychoogyl,* 106, 2, 243-250, 0021-843X

Dayas, C.V.; Liu, X.; Simms, J.A. & Weiss, F. (2007). Distinct patterns of neural activation associated with ethanol seeking: effects of naltrexone. *Biological Psychiatry,* 61, 8, 979-989, 0006-3223

De Vries, T.J. & Schoffelmeer, A.N.M. (2005). Cannabinoid CB1 receptors control conditioned drug seeking. *Trends in Pharmacological Sciences,* 26, 8, 420–426, 0165-6147

Di Chiara, G. (2002). Nucleus accumbens shell and core dopamine: differential role in behavior and addiction. *Behavioural Brain Research*, 137, 75-114, 0166-4328

Di Chiara, G. & Bassareo, V. (2007). Reward system and addiction: what dopamine does and doesn't do. *Current Opinion in Pharmacology*, 7, 1, 69-76, 1471-4892

Drummond, D.C. (2000). What does cue-reactivity have to offer clinical research? *Addiction*, 95, 8s2, 129- 144, 0965-2140

Drummond, D.C. & Glautier, S. (1994). A controlled trial of cue exposure treatment in alcohol dependence. *Journal of Consulting and Clinical Psychology*, 62, 4, 809–817, 0022-006X

Everitt, B.J. & Robbins, T.W. (2005). Neural systems of reinforcement for drug addiction: from actions to habits to compulsion. *Nature Neuroscience*, 8, 1481–1489, 1097-6256

Floresco, S.B.; Todd, C.L. & Grace, A.A. (2001). Glutamatergic afferents from the hippocampus to the nucleus accumbens regulate activity of ventral tegmental area dopamine neurons. The *Journal of Neuroscience*, 21, 4915-4922, 0270-6474

Fuster, J.M. (1997). *The Prefrontal Cortex: Anatomy, Physiology, and Neuropsychology of the Frontal Lobe*, Lippincott-Raven, 0397518498, Philadelphia.

George, M.S.; Anton, R.F.; Bloomer, C.; Teneback, C.; Drobes, D.J.; Lorberbaum, J.P.; Nahas, Z. & Vincent, D.J. (2001). Activation of prefrontal cortex and anterior thalamus in alcoholic subjects on exposure to alcohol-specific cues. *Archives of General Psychiatry*, 58, 4, 345–352, 0003-990x

George, D.T.; Gilman, J.; Hersh, J.; Thorsell, A.; Herion, D.; Geyer, C.; Peng, X.; Kielbasa, W.; Rawlings, R.; Brandt, J.E.; Gehlert, D.R.; Tauscher, J.T.; Hunt, S.P.; Hommer, D. & Heilig, M. (2008). Neurokinin 1 receptor antagonism as a possible therapy for alcoholism. *Science*, 319, *5869*, 1536-1539, 0036-8075

Gonzales, R.A. & Weiss, F. (1998). Suppression of ethanol-reinforced behavior by naltrexone is associated with attenuation of the ethanol-induced increase in dialysate dopamine levels in the nucleus accumbens. *The Journal of Neuroscience*, 18, 24, 10663–10671, 0270-6474

Goto, Y. & Grace, A.A. (2005). Dopamine-dependent interactions between limbic and prefrontal cortical synaptic plasticity in the nucleus accumbens: Disruption by cocaine sensitization. *Neuron*, 47, 2, 255-266, 0896-6273

Grüsser, S.M.; Wrase, J.; Klein, S.; Hermann, D.; Smolka, M.N.; Ruf, M.; Weber-Fahr, W.; Flor, H.; Mann, K.; Braus, D.F. & Heinz, A. (2004). Cue-induced activation of the striatum and medial prefrontal cortex is associated with subsequent relapse in abstinent alcoholics. *Psychopharmacology (Berl)*, 175, 3, 296–302, 0033-3158

Heinz, A.; Dufeu, P.; Kuhn, S.; Dettling, M.; Gräf, K.; Kürten, I.; Rommelspacher, H. & Schmidt, L.G. (1996). Psychopathological and behavioral correlates of dopaminergic sensitivity in alcohol dependent patients. *Archives of General Psychiatry*, 53:1123–1128, 0003-990x

Heinz, A.; Jones, D.W.; Zajicek, K.; Gorey, J.G.; Juckel, G.; Higley, J.D. & Weinberger, D.R. (2004a). Depletion and restoration of endogenous monoamines affects β-CIT binding to serotonin but not dopamine transporters in non-human primates. *Journal of Neural Transmission*, 68 (Suppl), 29-38, 0300-9564

Heinz, A.; Löber, S.; Georgi, A.; Wrase, J.; Hermann, D.; Rey, E.R.; Wellek, S. & Mann, K. (2003). Reward craving and withdrawal relief craving: assessment of different motivational pathways to alcohol intake. *Alcohol and Alcoholism,* 38, 1, 35–39, 0735-0414

Heinz, A.; Reimold, M.; Wrase, J.; Hermann, D.; Croissant, B.; Mundle, G.; Dohmen, B.M.; Braus, D.F.; Schumann, G.; Machulla, H.J.; Bares, R. & Mann, K. (2005a). Correlation of stable elevations in striatal μ-opioid receptor availability in detoxified alcoholic patients with alcohol craving–A positron emission tomography study using carbon 11-labeled carfentanil. *Archives of General Psychiatry,* 62, 1, 57-64, 0003-990x

Heinz, A.; Siessmeier, T.; Wrase, J.; Buchholz, H.G.; Gründer, G.; Kumakura, Y.; Cumming, P.; Schreckenberger, M.; Smolka, M.N.; Rösch, F.; Mann, K. & Bartenstein, P. (2005b). Correlation of alcohol craving with striatal dopamine synthesis capacity and D-2/3 receptor availability: a combined [18F]DOPA and [18F]DMFP PET Study in detoxified alcoholic patients. *The American Journal of Psychiatry,* 162, 1515–1520, 0002-953X

Heinz, A.; Siessmeier, T.; Wrase, J.; Hermann, D.; Klein, S.; Grüsser, S.M.; Flor, H.; Braus, D.F.; Buchholz, H.G.; Gründer, G.; Schreckenberger, M.; Smolka, M.N.; Rösch, F.; Mann, K. & Bartenstein, P. (2004b). Correlation between dopamine D-2 receptors in the ventral striatum and central processing of alcohol cues and craving. *The American Journal of Psychiatry,* 161, 1783–1789, 0002-953X

Heinz, A.; Wrase, J.; Kahnt, T.; Beck, A.; Bromand, Z.; Grüsser, S.M.; Kienast, T.; Smolka, M.N.; Flor, H. & Mann, K. (2007). Brain activation elicited by affectively positive stimuli is associated with a lower risk of relapse in detoxified alcoholic subjects. *Alcoholism: Clinical and Experimental Research,* 31, 7, 1138-1147, 0145-6008

Hermann, D.; Smolka, M.N.; Wrase, J.; Klein, S.; Nikitopoulos, J.; Georgi, A.; Braus, D.F.; Flor, H.; Mann, K. & Heinz, A. (2006). Blockade of cue-induced brain activation of abstinent alcoholics by a single administration of amisulpride as measured with fMRI. *Alcoholism: Clinical and Experimental Research,* 30, 1349-1354, 0145-6008

Hyman, S.E. & Malenka, R.C. (2001). Addiction and the brain: the neurobiology of compulsion and its persistence. *Nature Review Neuroscience,* 2, 10, 695–703, 1471-003X

Hyman, S.E. (2005). Addiction: A Disease of Learning and Memory. *American Journal of Psychiatry,* 162, 8, 1414–1422, 0002-953X

Junghanns, K.; Tietz, U.; Dibbelt, L.; Kuether, M.; Jurth, R.; Ehrenthal, D.; Blank, S. & Backhaus, J. (2005). Attenuated salivary cortisol secretion under cue exposure is associated with early relapse. *Alcohol and Alcoholism,* 40, 1, 80–85, 0735-0414

Kalivas, P.W. & Volkow, N.D. (2005). The neural basis of addiction: a pathology of motivation and choice. *American Journal of Psychiatry,* 162, 8, 1403–1413, 0002-953X

Kalivas, P.W.; Volkow, N. & Seamans, J. (2005). Unmanageable motivation in addiction: a pathology in prefrontal-accumbens glutamate transmission. *Neuron,* 45, 5, 647–650, 0896-6273

Kauer, J.A. (2004). Learning mechanisms in addiction: synaptic plasticity in the ventral tegmental area as a result of exposure to drugs of abuse. *Annual Review of Physiology,* 66, 447–475, 0066-4278

Kavanagh, D.J.; Andrade, J. & May, J. (2004). Beating the urge: implications of research into substance-related desires. *Addictive Behaviors,* 29, 7, 1359–1372, 0306-4603

Kiefer, F.; Helwig, H.; Tarnaske, T.; Otte, C.; Jahn, H. & Wiedemann, K. (2005). Pharmacological relapse prevention of alcoholism: clinical predictors of outcome. *European Addiction Research*, 11, 2, 83–91, 1022-6877

Kienast, T.; Siessmeier, T.; Wrase, J.; Braus, D.F.; Smolka, M.N.; Buchholz, H.G.; Rapp, M.; Schreckenberger, M.; Rösch, F.; Cumming, P.; Gruender, G.; Mann, K.; Bartenstein, P. & Heinz, A. (2008). Ratio of dopamine synthesis capacity to D_2-receptor availability in ventral striatum correlates with central processing of affective stimuli. *European Journal of Nuclear Medicine and Molecular Imaging*, 35, 6, 1147-1158, 1619-7070

Koob, G.F. (2003). Alcoholism: Allostasis and beyond. *Alcoholism, Clinical and Experimental Research*, 27, 2, 232-243, 0145-6008

Krystal, J.H.; Staley, J.; Mason, G.; Petrakis, I.L.; Kaufman, J.; Harris, R.A.; Gelernter, J. & Lappalainen, J. (2006). Gamma-aminobutyric acid type A receptors and alcoholism: intoxication, dependence, vulnerability, and treatment. *Archives of General Psychiatry*, 63, 9, 957-968, 0003-990X

Kumakura, Y.; Cumming, P.; Vernaleken, I.; Buchholz, H.G.; Siessmeier, T.; Heinz, A.; Kienast, T.; Bartenstein, P. & Gründer, G (2007). Elevated [18F]fluorodopamine turnover in brain of patients with schizophrenia: An [18F]fluorodopa/positron emissiontomography study. *Journal of Neuroscience*, 27, 30, 8080-8087, 0270-6474

Kwong, K.K.; Belliveau, J.W.; Chesler, D.A.; Goldberg, I.E.; Weisskoff, R.M.; Poncelet, B.P.; Kennedy, D.N.; Hoppel, B.E.; Cohen, M.S.; Turner, R.; Cheng, H.; Brady, T.J. & Rosen, B.R. (1992). Dynamic Magnetic Resonance Imaging of Human Brain Activity During Primary Sensory Stimulation. *PNAS*, 89, 12; 5675-5679, 0027-8424

Laruelle, M. (2000). Imaging synaptic neurotransmission with in vivo binding competition techniques: A critical review. *Journal of Cerebral Blood Flow and Metabolism*, 20, 423-451, 0271-678X

Lisman, J.E. & Grace, A.A. (2005). The hippocampal-VTA loop: Controlling the entry of information into long-term memory. *Neuron*, 46, 5, 703–713, 0896-6273

Litt, M.D.; Cooney, N.L. & Morse, P. (2000). Reactivity to alcohol-related stimuli in the laboratory and in the field: Predictors of craving in treated alcoholics. *Addiction*, 95, 6, 889–900, 0965-2140

Löber, S.; Croissant, B.; Heinz, A.; Mann, K. & Flor, H. (2006). Cue exposure in the treatment of alcohol dependence: Effects on drinking outcome, craving and self-efficacy. *British Journal of Clinical Psychology*, 45, 4, 515-529, 0144-6657

Lodge, D.J. & Grace, A.A. (2008). Augmented hippocampal drive of mesolimbic dopamine neurons: A mechanism of psychostimulant sensitization. *Journal of Neuroscience*, 28, 31, 7876-7882, 0270-6474

Logothetis, N.K. (2002) The neural basis of the blood-oxygen-level-dependent functional magnetic resonance imaging signal. *Philosophical transactions of the Royal Society of London. Series B, Biological sciences,* 357, 1424, 1003-1037, 1471-2970

Ludwig, A.M. & Wikler, A. (1974). Craving and relapse to drink. *Quarterly journal of Studies on Alcohol*, 35, 1-A, 108–130, 0033-5649

Mann, K.; Lehert, P. & Morgan, M.Y. (2004). The efficacy of acamprosate in the maintenance of abstinence in alcohol-dependent individuals: Results of a meta-analysis. *Alcoholism, Clinical and Experimental Research*, 28, 1, 51–63, 0145-6008

Martinez, D.; Gil, R.; Slifstein, M.; Hwang, D.R.; Huang, Y.; Perez, A.; Kegeles, L.; Talbot, P.; Evans, S.; Krystal, J.; Laruelle, M. & Abi-Dargham, A. (2005). Alcohol dependence is associated with blunted dopamine transmission in the ventral striatum. *Biological Psychiatry*, 58, 10, 779–786, 0006-3223

Modell, J.G. & Mountz, J.M. (1995). Focal cerebral blood flow change during craving for alcohol measured by SPECT. *The Journal of Neuropsychiatry and Clinical Neurosciences*, 7, 1, 15–22, 0895-0172

Monti, P.M.; Abrams, D.B.; Binkoff, J.A.; Zwick, W.R.; Liepman, M.R.; Nirenberg, T.D. & Rohsenow, D.J. (1990). Communication skills training, communication skills training with family and cognitive behavioural mood management-training for alcoholics. *Journal of Studies on Alcohol*, 51, 3, 263–270, 0096-882X

Myrick, H.; Anton, R.F.; Li, X.B.; Henderson, S.; Drobes, D.; Voronin, K. & George, M.S. (2004). Differential brain activity in alcoholics and social drinkers to alcohol cues: relationship to craving. *Neuropsychopharmacology*, 29, 2, 393–402, 0893-133X

Myrick, H.; Anton, R.F.; Li, X.; Henderson, S.; Randall, P.K. & Voronin, K. (2008). Effect of naltrexone and ondansetron on alcohol cue-induced activation of the ventral striatum in alcohol-dependent people. *Archives of General Psychiatry*. 65, 4, 466-475, 0003-990X

O'Brien, C.P. (2005). Anticraving medications for relapse prevention: A possible new class of psychoactive medications. *American Journal of Psychiatry*, 162, 8, 1423–1431, 0002-953X

Ogawa, S.; Lee, T.M.; Nayak, A.S. & Glynn, P. (1990). Oxygenation-sensitive contrast in magnetic resonance image of rodent brain at high magnetic fields. *Magnetic Resonance in Medicine*, 14, 1, 68-78, 0740-3194

Paulus, M.P.; Tapert, S.F. & Schuckit, M.A. (2005). Neural activation patterns of methamphetamine-dependent subjects during decision making predict relapse. *Archives of General Psychiatry*, 62, 7, 761-768, 0003-990X

Park, S.Q.; Kahnt, T.; Beck, A.; Cohen, M.X.; Dolan, R.J.; Wrase, J. & Heinz, A. (2010). Prefrontal cortex fails to learn from reward prediction errors in alcohol dependence. Journal of Neuroscience, 30, 22, 7749-7753, 0270-6474

Robbins, T.W. & Everitt, B.J. (2002). Limbic-striatal memory systems and drug addiction. *Neurobiology of learning and memory*, 78, 3, 625-636, 1074-7427

Robinson, T.E. & Berridge, K.C. (1993). The neural basis of drug craving–an incentive-sensitization theory of addiction. Brain research. Brain research reviews , 18, 3, 247–291, 0165-0173

Robinson, T,E. & Kolb, B. (1997). Persistent structural modifications in nucleus accumbens and prefrontal cortex neurons produced by previous experience with amphetamine. *Journal of Neuroscience*, 17, 21, 8491–8497, 0270-6474

Rohsenow, D.J.; Monti, P.M.; Rubonis, A.V.; Sirota, A.D.; Niaura, R.S.; Colby, S.M.; Wunschel, S.M. & Abrams, D.B. (1994). Cue reactivity as a predictor of drinking among male alcoholics. *Journal of Consulting and Clinical Psychology*, 62, 3, 620–626, 0022-006X

Rossetti, Z.L.; Melis, F.; Carboni, S. & Gessa, G.L. (1992). Dramatic depletion of mesolimbic extracellular dopamine after withdrawal from morphine, alcohol or cocaine–a common neurochemical substrate for drug-dependence. *Annals of the New York Academy of Sciences*, 654, 513–516, 0077-8923

Schneider, F.; Habel, U.; Wagner, M.; Franke, P.; Salloum, J.B.; Shah, N.J.; Toni, I.; Sulzbach, C.; Hönig, K.; Maier, W.; Gaebel, W. & Zilles, K. (2001). Subcortical correlates of craving in recently abstinent alcoholic patients. *American Journal of Psychiatry*, 158, 7, 1075–1083, 0002-953X

Schultz, W.; Dayan, P. & Montague, P.R. (1997). A neural substrate of prediction and reward. *Science*, 275, 1593–1599, 0193-4511

Schumann, G.; Saam, C.; Heinz, A.; Mann, K. & Treutlein, J. (2005). The NMDA receptor system: Genetic risk factor for alcoholism. *Nervenarzt*, 76, 11, 1355-1362, 0028-2804

Shalev, U.; Grimm, J.W. & Shaham, Y. (2002). Neurobiology of relapse to heroin and cocaine seeking: a review. *Pharmacological Reviews*, 54, 1, 1–42, 0031-6997

Shalev, U.; Highfield, D.; Yap, J. & Shaham, Y. (2000). Stress and relapse to drug seeking in rats: Studies on the generality of the effect. *Psychopharmacology*, 150, 3, 337-46, 0033-3158

Siegel, S. (1975). Evidence from rats that morphinetolerance is a learned response. *Journal of comparative and physiological psychology*, 89, 5, 498–506, 0021-9940

Siegel, S.; Hinson, R.E.; Krank, M.D. & Mccully, J. (1982). Heroin Overdose Death - Contribution of Drug-Associated Environmental Cues. *Science*, 216, 4544, 436-437, 0193-4511

Spanagel, R. (2003). The role of the glutamatergic system in alcohol addiction. *Fortschritte der Neurologie-Psychiatrie*, 71, S33–S35, 0720-4299

Srisurapanont, M. & Jarusuraisin, N. (2005). Naltrexone for the treatment of alcoholism: A meta-analysis of randomized controlled trials. *International Journal of Neuropsychopharmacology*, 8, 2, 267–280, 1461-1457

Tapert, S.F.; Brown, G.G.; Baratta, M.V. & Brown, S.A. (2004). FMRI BOLD response to alcohol stimuli in alcohol dependent young women. *Addictive Behaviors*, 29, 1, 33–50, 0306-4603

Tiffany, S.T. (1990). A cognitive model of drug urges and drug-use behavior–role of automatic and nonautomatic processes. *Psychological Review*, 97, 2, 147–168, 0033-295X

Thomas, M.J. & Malenka, R.C. (2003). Synaptic plasticity in the mesolimbic dopamine system. *Philosophical transactions of the Royal Society of London. Series B, Biological sciences*, 358, 1432, 815–819, 1471-2970

Tobler, P.N.; Fiorillo, C.D. & Schultz, W. (2005). Adaptive coding of reward value by dopamine neurons. *Science*, 307, 5715, 1642–1645, 0193-4511

Tsai, G.; Gastfriend, D.R. & Coyle, J.T. (1995). The glutamatergic basis of human alcoholism. *American Journal of Psychiatry*, 152, 3, 332-40, 0002-953X

Vanderschuren L.J.; Di Ciano, P. & Everitt, B.J. (2005). Involvement of the dorsal striatum in cue-controlled cocaine seeking. *Journal of Neuroscience*, 25, 38, 8665–8670, 0270-6474

Verheul, R.; van den Brink, W. & Geerlings, P. (1999). A three-pathway psychobiological model of craving for alcohol. *Alcohol and Alcoholism*, 34, 2, 197-222, 0735-0414

Volkow, N.D.; Fowler, J.S.; Wang, G.J. & Swanson, J.M. (2004). Dopamine in drug abuse and addiction: results from imaging studies and treatment implications. *Molecular Psychiatry*, 9, 557-69, 1359-4184

Volkow, N.D.; Wang, G.J.; Fowler, J.S.; Logan, J.; Hitzemann, R.; Ding, Y.S.; Pappas, N.; Shea C. & Piscani, K. (1996). Decreases in dopamine receptors but not in dopamine transporters in alcoholics. *Alcohol: Clinical and Experimental Research*, 20, 9, 1594–1598, 0145-6008

Volkow, N.D.; Wang, G.J.; Telang, F.; Fowler, J.S.; Logan, J.; Childress, A.R.; Jayne, M.; Ma, Y. & Wong, C. (2006). Cocaine cues and dopamine in dorsal striatum: Mechanism of craving in cocaine addiction. *Journal of Neuroscience*, 26, 24, 6583-6588, 0270-6474

Vorel, S.R.; Liu, X.; Hayes, R.J.; Spector, J.A. & Gardner, E.L. (2001). Relapse to cocaine-seeking after hippocampal theta burst stimulation. *Science*, 292, 5519, 1175–1178, 0193-4511

Wikler, A. (1948). Recent Progress in Research on the Neurophysiologic Basis of Morphine Addiction. *American Journal of Psychiatry*, 105, 329-338, 0002-953X

Wise, R.A. (1988). The neurobiology of craving: implications for the understanding and treatment of addiction. *Journal of Abnormal Psychology*, 97, 2, 118-132, 0021-843X

Wong, D.F.; Kuwabara, H.; Schretlin, D.; Bonson, K.; Zhou, Y.; Nandi, A.; Brasic, J.; Kimes A.S.; Maris, M.A.; Kumar, A.; Contoreggi, C.; Links, J.; Ernst, M.; Rousset, O.; Zukin, S.; Grace, A.A.; Rohde, C.; Jasinski, D.R.; Gjedde, A. & London, E.D. (2006). Increased occupancy of dopamine receptors in human striatum during cue-elicited cocaine craving. *Neuropsychopharmacology*, 31, 2716-2727, 0893-133X

World Health Organization (2007). *International Statistical Classification of Diseases and Related Problems*, World Health Organization, 9241546530, Geneva

Wrase, J.; Grüsser, S.M.; Klein, S.; Diener, C.; Hermann, D.; Flor, H.; Mann, K.; Braus, D.F. & Heinz, A. (2002). Development of alcohol-associated cues and cue-induced brain activation in alcoholics. *European Psychiatry*, 17, 5, 287–291, 0924-9338

Wrase, J.; Schlagenhauf, F.; Kienast, T.; Wüstenberg, T.; Bermpohl, F.; Kahnt, T.; Beck, A.; Ströhle, A.; Juckel, G.; Knutson, B. & Heinz, A. (2007). Dysfunction of reward processing correlates with alcohol craving in detoxified alcoholics. *Neuroimage*, 35, 2, 787-794, 1053-8119

6

Clinical Magnetic Resonance Neuroimaging in Fibromyalgia

Nicolás Fayed* and Javier Garcia-Campayo**

*Department of Radiology, Quirón Hospital, Zaragoza, Spain**

*Somatoform Disorders and Fibromyalgia Unit, Miguel Servet Hospital, University of Zaragoza, Spain***

Key points

- Magnetic resonance spectroscopy (MRS) offers invaluable information about living tissues with special contribution to the diagnosis and prognosis of the central nervous system diseases.
- Diffusion tensor imaging (DTI) detects subtle degradation of white matter microstructure in fibromyalgia.
- Perfusion magnetic resonance imaging (MRI) offers higher spatial resolution than radionuclide techniques such as positron emission tomography and single-photon emission computed tomography.
- Voxel-based morphometry (VBM) is a recent methodology that can simultaneously visualize group differences or statistical effects on gray and white matter, throughout the whole brain.
- Functional magnetic resonance imaging (fMRI) studies regularly confirm that multiple brain regions are invoked to execute even ostensibly simple tasks.

1. Introduction

Imaging human internal organs with exact and non-invasive methods is very important in medicine for medical diagnosis, treatment and follow-up, as well as for clinical research. Today, one of the most important tools for this purpose is magnetic resonance imaging (MRI). MRI scanners are based on the nuclear magnetic resonance (NMR) phenomenon, which was detected independently by Bloch, Purcell et al. in 1946. The advent of neuroimaging techniques yielding neuropsychological data in addition to structural information was of particular interest for scientific and clinical research into fibromyalgia and psychiatric disorders. These are groups of conditions for which any structural changes evident in anatomical imaging sequences generally correlate poorly with clinical diagnostic categories, pointing to underlying pathophysiology and severity of disease. T1- and T2-dependent MR sequences, the mainstay of routine clinical neuroimaging, are frequently insensitive to the underlying pathological processes in these conditions. Focal or global atrophy due to associated neuronal loss is also frequently absent.

The remit of this section is an overview of some general issues concerning the application of spectroscopy, diffusion, perfusion, morphometry and functional techniques in fibromyalgia, and their clinical impact in the context of other available tests.

2. Magnetic Resonance Spectroscopy (MRS)

This technique enables us to study the chemical composition of living tissues. It is based on the chemical shift of atoms. The concentration of some metabolites is determined from spectra that may be acquired in several ways.

3. Voxel placement

Currently the spectra may be acquired with single-voxel (SV) or multivoxel techniques (MV). The SV technique is readily available on most scanners. Voxels must be positioned away from sources of susceptibility artifacts and lipids. For diffuse processes, a 2 x 2 x 2-cm (8 cm3) voxel is routinely used. For local lesions, the SV can be reduced in volume. The SV technique offers the advantages of better spatial location, more homogeneity, better water suppression and speed. However, only one spectrum can be obtained per acquisition.
However, The MV technique makes it possible to obtain multiple spectra simultaneously per acquisition and to assess a greater area of the brain but with smaller spectral resolution. To date, the SV is still superior to MV on the grounds of reproducibility (Sauter et al., 1991; Hsu et al., 1999, 2001; Law et al., 2004). For both SV and MV, the MR scanner employs a process known as shimming to narrow peak linewidths within the spectra. For SV studies, improving field homogeneity is performed with basic, zero-ordered shimming on clinical MR scanners. For MV, the simultaneous production of uniform field homogeneity in multiple regions requires higher order shimming. To obtain high-quality spectra, blood products, air, fat, necrotic areas, cerebrospinal fluid, metal, calcification and bone should be avoided. In such areas differing magnetic susceptibility results in a non-homogenous field that hinders the production of diagnostic quality spectra.

4. MRS pulse sequence

Two different approaches are generally used for proton spectroscopy of the brain: a) single-voxel methods based on the stimulated echo acquisition mode (STEAM) and b) point resolved spectroscopy (PRESS) pulse sequences and spectroscopy imaging (SI), also known as chemical shift imaging (CSI). These latter studies are usually done in two dimensions, using a variety of different pulse sequences (spin-echo (SE), usually PRESS).
The basic principle underlying single-voxel localization techniques is to use three mutually orthogonal slice selective pulses and design the pulse sequence to collect only the echo signal from the point (voxel) in space where all three slices intersect. In STEAM, three 90° pulses are used and the stimulated echo is collected. All other signals (echoes) should be dephased by the large crusher gradient applied during the so-called mixing time. Crusher gradients are necessary for consistent formation of the stimulated echo and removal of unwanted coherences. In PRESS, the second and third pulses are refocusing (180°) pulses, and crusher gradients are applied around these pulses to select the desired SE signal arising

from all three RF pulses and dephasing unwanted coherences. STEAM and PRESS are generally similar but differ in a few key aspects.
With regard to the mode of acquisition, PRESS can be performed with short and long echo times (TEs) and there is complete recovery of signal. STEAM can be performed with very short TEs, but there is incomplete recovery of signal and a precise volume element (voxel) is formed. The PRESS mode is used more than STEAM because it increases the signal/noise ratio and is less sensitive to movement artifacts (Maheshwari et al. 2000). A short TE (20-40 ms) allows us to increase the signal/noise ratio and to visualize most metabolite peaks, with the inconvenience of some degree of peak overlapping of. Time matters in clinical practice, so short TEs are preferable. In our experience with a 1.5T GE Signa Horizon-clinical scanner a TE of 30 ms and a TR of 2500 ms have proven valuable (Fayed et al., 2006). Recently, a TE-averaged PRESS technique has been yielding highly simplified spectra with better suppression of signals not pertaining to assessed metabolites, such as that of macromolecules. TE is increased from 35 ms to 355 ms in steps of 2.5 ms with two acquisitions per step (Hancu et al., 2005).

5. MR spectra quantification

The most commonly used spectroscopy is that originating from a Hydrogen nucleus (proton 1H-MRS). This technique is based on the differences in resonance obtained from hydrogen nuclei depending on the surrounding atoms (chemical shift). Each metabolite being assessed discloses a different hydrogen resonance frequency and appears in a different site in the spectrum. The most frequently evaluated metabolites are N-acetyl-aspartate (NAA), myo-inositol (mI), choline (Ch), creatine (Cr) and glutamate+glutamine (Glx). The position of the metabolite signal is identified on the horizontal axis by its chemical shift, scaled in units referred to as parts per million (ppm). With the appropriate factors considered, such as the number of protons, relaxation times and so forth, a signal can be converted into a metabolite concentration by measuring the area under the curve. Because water is the main component of living beings and its concentration is much higher than that of metabolites, it becomes necessary to suppress the resonance signal from the hydrogen of water (Maheshwari et al. 2000 and Bonavita et al. 1999). A plot showing peak amplitudes and frequencies is obtained. Each spectrum shows peaks corresponding to the different metabolite values: Myo-inositol (mI), 3.56 and 4.06 ppm; Choline compounds (Ch), 3.23 ppm; Creatine (Cr), 3.03 and 3.94 ppm; y N-acetil-aspartate (NAA), 2.02; 2.5 and 2.6 ppm; glutamine and glutamate (Glx), 2.1-2.55 ppm and 3.8 ppm . Ratios between metabolites and creatine are also of great value as they counteract the systematic errors of measurements.

6. Fitting of model spectra

A more recent program, called a linear combination model ("LCModel") (Provencher, 1993), fits in vivo spectra as a linear superposition of high-resolution "basis" spectra that are acquired from model solutions of the metabolites present in the organ of interest. Advantages of LCModel are that all pre-processing steps, automatic phase correction as well as modelling of a smooth baseline are included. Standardized basis sets are available for the most common clinical MR machines (both 1.5 and 3 T).

7. Fibromyalgia

Fibromyalgia is a chronic and disabling musculoskeletal pain disorder of unknown, characterized by a history of widespread pain for at least three months and patients reporting of tenderness in at least 11 of 18 defined tender points when digitally palpated with about 4 kg per unit area of force. Other frequent accompanying symptoms are fatigue, sleep disturbance and depressed mood (Wolfe et al, 1990; Giesecke et al, 2003). With an estimated lifetime prevalence of 2% in community samples (Wolfe et al, 1995), it accounts for 15% of outpatient rheumatology visits and 5% of primary care visits (Wolfe 1989). The prognosis for symptomatic recovery is generally poor (Wolfe et al., 1997). Recent meta-analysis (Garcia Campayo et al., 2008) demonstrates that both pharmacological and psychological treatments show moderate effectiveness with a mean effect size of 0.49. The variables that related most with improvement in outcome were younger age of the patients and shorter duration of the disorder. On the contrary, gender and type of treatment (pharmacological or psychological) did not affect outcome (Garcia Campayo et al., 2008).

8. Usefulness of different neuroimaging techniques in Fibromyalgia

a) 1H MRS in Fibromyalgia patients

Glutamate has been implicated as an important mediator in the neurotransmission, potentiation, and negative affect associated with pain, and it has been related to chronic pain sensitization (Dickenson et al., 2002). Experimental pain models for fibromyalgia have revealed elevated glutamate levels in the posterior insula. MRS spectroscopy studies have shown that dynamic changes in glutamate and glutamine levels in the insula were associated with improvements in clinical and experimental pain in fibromyalgia (Harris et al., 2008). Also, a recent MR spectroscopy study concludes with the involvement of the posterior insula in pain (Harris et al., 2009)

A previous MRS study by our group demonstrated the differences in metabolites between FM patients and controls. (A)

Our data suggest that Glx plays a role in this augmented pain processing in those individuals who have elevated Glx levels, which is entirely consistent with the literature and knowledge regarding FM. In our study there is a significant correlation in the posterior cingulate gyrus between Glu+Gln (Glx) and Glx/Cr with depression, pain measured in an objective way, such as by sphygmomanometer, and global function assessed with the Fybromyalgia Impact Questionnaire (FIQ). Since astrocytes participate in the uptake, metabolism, and recycling of glutamate, we hypothesize that an astrocyte deficit may account for the alterations in glutamate/GABA neurotransmission in depression. Factors such as stress, excess glucocorticoids, altered gene expression of neurotrophic factors and glial transporters, and changes in extracellular levels of neurotransmitters released by neurons may modify glial cell numbers and affect the neurophysiology of depression (Rajkowska et al., 2007). Other studies found that absolute concentrations of Glx, Glu, and creatine+phosphocreatine (Cr) were significantly higher in adult bipolar patients in all mood states compared to healthy controls (Yildiz-Yesiloglu et al. 2006).

Elevated Glx inside the astrocyte leads to increased cellular osmolarity in the brain. Within 30 minutes of glutamate administration, electron microscopy reveals massive acute swelling of neuronal cell bodies and dendrites. Consequently, water shifts from the extracellular fluid space to the intracellular fluid space resulting in edema of the astrocytes. Relevant clinical manifestations are thought to be secondary to this edema (Häussinger et al., 2000). To compensate for the increased cellular osmolarity, myo-inositol shifts to the extracellular fluids space, leading to a reduction in its concentration inside the astrocyte. In consequence, Glx is an excitatory amino acid, and its increase indicates that the metabolic function of patients with fibromyalgia differs from controls. Elevation of Gln levels may result in permanent cerebral damage.

In addition, high correlations were found between some clinical variables and certain brain metabolites, for instance: ratios of myo-Inositol/Creatine and NAA + *N*-acetyl aspartyl glutamate (NAA+NAAG) in the left hippocampus with pain; myo-Inositol in the right hippocampus and myo-Inositol in the posterior cingulate gyrus with catastrophization.

A recent HMRS study, showed decreased NAA levels within the hippocampus of individuals with FM (Wood et al., 2009). In another study, a reduction in the absolute concentration of NAA in the right and left hippocampi was reported in a sample of 15 patients with fibromyalgia (Emad et al. 2008). Lower hippocampal NAA levels suggest neuronal or axonal metabolic dysfunction, or some combination of these processes. Neuronal loss in the hippocampus has not yet been studied in our series. This should be assessed in further studies, in order to gauge atrophic changes within the hippocampus. Some studies found that the persistence of elevated Ca2+ in hippocampal neurons exposed to glutamate correlated with the extent of neuronal death, and that a large rise in Ca2+ in cultured hippocampal neurons, following glutamate application, predicted cell death (Mattson et al., 1989). Hippocampal dysfunction may be partly responsible for some of the phenomena associated with FM. Blocking NMDA receptors in the hippocampal formation reduces nociceptive behaviours; this in turn supports the hypothesis that the hippocampal formation is involved in pain-related neural processing and expression of pain-related behaviours (McKenna et al. 2001).

Finally, our study confirms the reduction in myo-Inositol levels in both hippocampi and reduction in myo-Inositol/Cr ratios in the left hippocampus and sensitivomotrice area. In all cases, brain metabolites were lower in the patient group compared to controls. Changes in myo-Inositol have previously been described in patients suffering from bipolar disorder (Silverstone et al. 2005). Research suggests that lithium functions primarily by decreasing myo-inositol concentrations in bipolar patients (Harwood et al., 2005).

Patients suffering from clinical depression generally have decreased levels of inositol in their cerebrospinal fluid (Barkai et al., 1978). This deficiency could be explained by a reduced synthesis or more interestingly by an increased consumption of the compound (Lentner, 1986). We speculate that myo-Inositol might, via its conversion to glucuronic acid, be consumed in protective detoxification reactions of the brain and could be associated with depression.

b) Diffusion Tensor Imaging (DTI)

White matter structure

Neuroimaging reveals changes in the white matter (WM) structure in the human brain. White matter comprises half of the human brain and consists of bundles of myelinated axons connecting neurons in different brain regions (Fields, 2008). Grey matter is composed of neuronal cell bodies and dendrites concentrated in the outer layers of the cortex. Microstructural changes in white matter can be revealed by specialized MRI brain imaging techniques such as diffusion tensor imaging (DTI). This method analyses the of proton diffusion in tissue, which is more restricted in white matter than in grey matter. The anisotropy increases with increased myelination, diameter and axon compaction.

DTI measurement

Water molecules in the brain are in constant Brownian motion, and although the movement of theses protons affects conventional structural imaging, diffusion weighted imaging (DWI) and diffusion tensor imaging (DTI) allow quantification of this microscopic movement within each voxel. The main advantage of using DTI, rather than DWI, is that DTI reflects the underlying diffusion properties of the sample, independently of the orientation of the tissue with respect to the direction of measurements. DTI is thus a robust quantitative technique that is independent of how the subject has been oriented inside the scanner magnet and gradient coils. In regions with few or no constraints imposed by physical boundaries, such as CSF in the ventricles, water movement is random in every direction and is isotropic. In contrast to CSF, the path of a water molecule in a WM fibre is constrained by physical boundaries, such as the axon sheath, causing the movement along the long axis of a fibre to be greater than radial diffusion across the.

These data can be used to calculate the probable anatomy of white matter bundles in living brain, a process called tractography. Orientation is calculated from the eigenvectors defining proton diffusion in three dimensions in each voxel. Using algorithms, the principal eigenvalue vector is connected to the next voxel to trace the fibre structure and orientation in white matter tracts (Jones et al., 2002)

Diffusion tensor imaging (DTI) yields quantitative measures for tissue water mobility as a function of the direction of water motion and is probed by application of diffusion-sensitization gradients in multiple directions (Basser et al., 1996). Basser et al. describe the use of multivariate linear regression to calculate D from a non-diffusion-weighted image plus six or more diffusion-weighted measurements in a non-collinear direction. The diffusion weighting is obtained by simultaneously applying diffusion gradients along combinations of the three physical axes.

The appropriate mathematical combination of the directional diffusion-weighted images provides quantitative measures of water diffusion for each voxel via the apparent diffusion coefficient (ADC), as well as the degree of diffusion directionality, or anisotropy (Sundgren et al. 2004). Myelin is a major diffusion barrier for water, and gives white matter its high anisotropy. Demyelinating diseases are characterized by partial or total loss of myelin, with consequent loss of neuronal function.

Fibromyalgia

DTI allows in vivo mapping of the anatomic connections in the human brain; previous studies have identified and confirmed the existence of an anatomic circuitry for the functionally characterized top-down influences on pain processing via brainstem structures in humans (Hadjipavlou et al., 2006) Fractional anisotropy (FA) is a measure of the portion of the diffusion tensor from anisotropy.

Previous studies with diffusion tensor imaging in FM patients showed alterations in the right thalamus and significantly lower fractionated anisotropy in comparison with controls. A negative correlation was seen between the FA values in the right thalamus and clinical pain in the FM group (Sundgren et al., 2007). Other authors confirmed that DTI in the brain of patients with FM appears to be more sensitive than volumetric imaging of voxel-based morphometry (VBM) and increased pain intensity scores were correlated with changes in DTI measurements in the right superior frontal gyrus. Increased fatigue was correlated with changes in the left superior frontal and left anterior cingulate gyrus, and self-perceived physical impairment was correlated with changes in the left postcentral gyrus. Higher intensity scores for stress symptoms were correlated negatively with diffusivity in the thalamus and FA in the left insular cortex (Lutz et al., 2008).

In a previous study by our group, DWI and DTI were not sensitive enough to detect changes in fibromyalgia patients. This may be explained because intraparenchymal injection of glutamate or other excitatory aminoacids cause neuronal cell bodies and dendrites to be predominantly affected, whereas axons and terminal boutons, originating from cell bodies outside of the affected region, remain largely intact (Coyle et al., 1981).

c) Perfusion MRI

Positron emission tomography (PET) (Jones et al., 1991) and single-photon emission computed tomography (SPECT) (Kwiatek et al., 2000) have been used to identify focal changes in regional cerebral blood flow (CBF) in patients with fibromyalgia. However, the low spatial resolution of PET and SPECT, and the ionizing radiation emitted from the nuclear medicine tracers are major concerns. MR perfusion techniques have also been developed and offer higher spatial resolution without the use of ionizing radiation (Rosen et al., 1990; Belliveau et al., 1990; Detre et al., 1992).

MR perfusion techniques are based on exogenous or endogenous tracers. In the method based on exogenous tracers, a paramagnetic agent such as gadolinium dimeglumine gadopentate (Gd-DTPA) is injected, and the resulting decrease and subsequent recovery of the MR signal is used to estimate perfusion (Ostergaard et al., 1996; Liu et al., 1999). In the method using endogenous tracers, the magnetization of the spins of arterial water are non-invasively labelled using radiofrequency (RF) pulses, and the regional accumulation of the label is measured in the tissues by comparison with an image acquired without labelling (Edelman et al., 1994; Kim, 1995; Kwong et al., 1995).

d) Voxel-based morphometry (VBM)

Tissue volumes in the CNS, and in particular changes in volume over time, are sensitive markers of a range of neurological disease states and disease progression. Measurement of brain volume requires segmentation of the brain from the rest of the tissues in the head and neck. Whilst this can be performed manually or in a semiautomated fashion (see for example Harris et al., 1999; Bokde et al., 2002), automated procedures are likely to be more reproducible and rapid. This is understandable as the size of the structures involved is usually relatively small, making the analysis less tedious than a manual segmentation of the whole brain. Additionally, many structures, such as the hippocampus, are difficult to segment in an automated fashion, but are relatively easily identified and manually or semiautomatically outlined, given appropriate software. Some progress has been made in automating segmentation procedures, with methods including the use of deformable shape models.

Tensor-based morphometry (TBM) is a relatively new image analysis technique that identifies regional structural differences in the brain, across groups or over time, from the gradients of the deformation fields that warp images to a common anatomical template. The anatomical information is encoded in the spatial transformation. Therefore, accurate inter-subject non-rigid registration is an essential tool. With the new advent of recent and powerful non-rigid registration algorithms based on the large deformation paradigm, TBM is being increasingly used (Lepore et al., 2008; Chiang et al., 2007; Lee et al., 2007).

In FM, Valet et al. (2009) found significant grey-matter decreases in the prefrontal, cingulate, and insular cortex. These regions are known to be critically involved in the modulation of subjective pain experiences. Patients presented a decrease in grey matter volume in the prefrontal cortex, the amygdala, and the anterior cingulate cortex (ACC). The duration of pain or functional pain disability did not correlate with grey matter volumes. A trend of inverse correlation of grey matter volume reduction in the ACC with the duration of pain medication intake has been detected. Some authors (Burgmer et al., 2009) suggest that structural changes in the pain system are associated with FM. As disease factors do not correlate with reduced grey matter volume in areas of the cingulo-frontal cortex and the amygdala in patients, one possible interpretation is that volume reductions might be a precondition for central sensitization in fibromyalgia.

e) Functional MR imaging (fMRI)

Another more recent imaging method is functional MRI (fMRI) for the mapping of activation patterns in the brain. This is an important technique for better understanding of brain function. When a brain region is activated, new energy must be transported to this region, which leads to increased blood flow to that part of the brain. This can be imaged by repetitive MR scans and detected by appropriate signal processing methods.

Over the years, many have viewed Fibromyalgia syndrome (FMS) as a so-called "functional disorder" and patients have experienced a concomitant lack of interest and legitimacy from the medical profession. The symptoms have not been explained by peripheral mechanisms alone or by specific central nervous system mechanisms.

Functional MRI blood oxygenation level dependent activation studies on patients who have FM have demonstrated augmented sensitivity to painful pressure and the association of this augmentation with variables such as depression and catastrophizing, and have also been used to evaluate the symptoms of cognitive dysfunction.

The fMRI-analysis by Jensen et al. (2009), revealed no differences in activity in brain regions related with attention and affection or regions with sensory projections from the stimulated body area. However, when there is a primary lesion in the descending pain regulating system (the rostral anterior cingulate cortex), the patients failed to respond to pain provocation. The attenuated response to pain in these cases is the first demonstration of a specific brain region where the impairment of pain inhibition in FMS patients is expressed. These results validate previous reports of dysfunctional endogenous pain inhibition in FM, and advance the understanding of the central pathophysiologic mechanisms, providing a new direction for the development of successful treatments in FM.

Fibromyalgia is the prototypical functional chronic pain condition, and it affects 2-4% of individuals. Although the aetiology of this disorder remains largely unknown, emerging data suggest that FM arises through augmentation of central pain processing pathways. This hypothesis is largely based upon findings of previous functional neuroimaging studies showing that FM patients display augmented neuronal responses to both innocuous and painful stimuli (Gracely et al., 2002; Cook et al., 2004), confirming the allodynia and hyperalgesia seen in this condition (Petzke et al., 2003).

Studies with functional neuroimaging support the hypothesis of central pain augmentation in FMS. Differences of activation in the fronto-cingulate cortex, the supplemental motor areas and the thalamus were found between both groups with distinct differences in BOLD-signals changes over the time course of pain stimulation, even during anticipation of pain. These results support the hypothesis that central mechanisms of pain processing in the medial pain system, favourable cognitive/affective factors even during the anticipation of pain, may play an important role for pain processing in patients with FMS (Burgmer et al., 2009).

9. Summary, conclusions and future directions

In this chapter, several techniques used for the diagnosis of fibromyalgia are discussed. At present, there are no other non-invasive techniques that can provide equivalent information and, as a consequence, MRS, DTI tractography and functional MRI are expected to be a powerful combined technique for researching brain anatomy and disease *in situ* in human beings.

Diffusion tensor imaging (DTI) in combination with magnetic resonance spectroscopy (MRS) and functional MRI (fMRI) may provide clinicians with information about ongoing pathological changes in FM. Future studies may investigate whether DTI can detect Many factors may influence the ability of DTI to discriminate patients with FM from healthy individuals. These factors include the field strength of the magnet, spatial resolution, signal-to-noise ratio, contrast-to-noise ratio and image artifacts. DTI and MRS are non-invasive and do not require the use of radioactive tracers, suggesting its potential safe application for longitudinal follow-up and repeated assessments.

Continued improvements in the design of imaging equipment and analysis algorithms are progressively improving the specificity of the biological parameters that can be calculated, allowing detailed quantitative characterization of microvascular structure in a wide range of pathological tissues, including fibromyalgia.

10. References

1. Barkai IA, Dunner DL, Gross HA, Mayo P, Fieve RR. Reduced myo-inositol levels in cerebrospinal fluid from patients with affective disorder. Biol Psychiatry 1978; 13: 65-72.
2. Basser PJ, Pierpaoli C. Microstructural and physiological features of tissues elucidated by quantitative-diffusion-tensor MRI. J Magn Reson B 1996; 111: 209-19.
3. Belliveau JW, Rosen BR, Kantor HL, Rzedzian RR, Kennedy DN, McKinstry RC, Vevea JM, Cohen MS, Pykett IL, Brady TJ. Functional cerebral imaging by susceptibility-contrast NMR. Magn Reson Med 1990; 14: 538-46.
4. Bloch F. Nuclear induction. Phys Rev 1946, 70:460-474.
5. Bonavita S, Di Salle F, Tedeschi G. Proton MRS in neurological disorders. Eur J Radiol 1999; 30: 125-31.
6. Burgmer M, Gaubitz M, Konrad C, Wrenger M, Hilgart S, Heuft G, Pfleiderer B. Decreased gray matter volumes in the cingulo-frontal cortex and the amygdala in patients with fibromyalgia. Psychosom Med 2009; 71: 566-73.

7. Burgmer M, Pogatzki-Zahn E, Gaubitz M, Wessoleck E, Heuft G, Pfleiderer B. Altered brain activity during pain processing in fibromyalgia. Neuroimage 2009; 44: 502-8.
8. Chiang MC, Dutton RA, Hayashi KM, Lopez OL, Aizenstein HJ, Toga AW, Becker JT, Thompson,PM: 3D pattern of brain atrophy in HIV/AIDS visualized using tensor-based morphometry. NeuroImage 2007; 34: 44–60.
9. Cook DB, Lange G, Ciccone DS, Liu WC, Steffener J, Natelson BH. Functional imaging of pain in patients with primary fibromyalgia. J Rheumatol 2004; 31: 364-78.
10. Coyle JT, Bird SJ, Evans RH, Gulley RL, Nadler JV, Nicjclas WJ, et al. Excitatory amino acid neurotoxins: selectively and mechanisms of action. Neurosci Res Prog 1981; 19: 1-427
11. Detre JA, Leigh JS, Williams DS, Koretsky AP. Perfusion imaging. Magn Reson Med. 1992; 23:37-45.
12. Edelman RR, Siewert B, Darby DG, Thangaraj V, Nobre AC, Mesulam MM, Warach S. Qualitative mapping of cerebral blood flow and functional localization with echo-planar MR imaging and signal targeting with alternating radio frequency. Radiology 1994; 192: 513-20.
13. Emad Y, Ragab Y, Zeinhom F, El-Khouly G, Abou-Zeid A, Rasker JJ. Hippocampus dysfunction may explain symptoms of fibromyalgia syndrome. A study with single-voxel magnetic resonance spectroscopy. J Rheumatol 2008; 35: 1371-7.
14. Fayed N, Morales H, Modrego PJ, Pina MA. Contrast/Noise ratio on conventional MRI and choline/creatine ratio on proton MRI spectroscopy accurately discriminate low-grade from high-grade cerebral gliomas. Acad Radiol 2006;13: 728-37.
15. Fayed N, Olmos S, Morales H, Modrego PJ. Physical Basis of Magnetic Resonance Spectroscopy and its Application to Central Nervous System Diseases. Am J Applied Sci 2006; 3:1836-1845.
16. Fields RD. White matter in learning, cognition and psychiatric disorders. Trends Neurosci 2008; 31: 317-376.
17. Hadjipavlou G, Dunckley P, Behrens TE, Tracey I. Determining anatomical connectivities between cortical and brainstem pain processing regions in humans: a diffusion tensor imaging study in healthy controls. Pain 2006; 123:169-78.
18. Hancu I, Zimmerman EA, Sailasuta N, Hurd RE. 1H MR spectroscopy using TE averaged PRESS: a more sensitive technique to detect neurodegeneration associated with Alzheimer's disease. Magn Reson Med 2005; 53:777-82.
19. Harris RE, Sundgren PC, Pang Y, Hsu M, Petrou M, Kim SH et al. Dynamic levels of glutamate within the insula are associated with improvements in multiple pain domains in fibromyalgia. Arthritis Rheum 2008; 58:903-7.
20. Harris RE, Sundgren PC, Craig AD, Kirshenbaum E, Sen A, Napadow V et al. Elevated insular glutamate in fibromyalgia is associated with experimental pain. Arthritis Rheum 2009; 60: 3146-52.
21. Harwood AJ. Lithium and bipolar mood disorder: the inositol-depletion hypothesis revisited. Mol Psychiatry 2005; 10: 117-26.
22. Häussinger D, Kircheis G, Fischer R, Schliess F, vom Dahl S. Hepatic encephalopathy in chronic liver disease: a clinical manifestation of astrocyte swelling and low-grade cerebral edema? J Hepatol 2000; 32: 1035-8.
23. Hsu YY, Chang C, Chang CN, Chu NS, Lim KE, Hsu JC. Proton MR spectroscopy in patients with complex partial seizures: single-voxel spectroscopy versus chemical-shift imaging. Am J Neuroradiol. 1999; 20(4): 643-51.

24. Hsu YY, Chen MC, Lim KE, Chang C. Reproducibility of hippocampal single-Voxel proton MR spectroscopy and chemical shift imaging. Am J Roentgenol 2001; 176: 529-36.
25. Garcia-Campayo J, Magdalena J, Magallón R, Fernández E, Salas M, Andrés E. A meta-analysis of the efficacy of fibromyalgia treatment according to level of care. Arthr Res Ther 2008; 10: R81.
26. Gracely RH, Petzke F, Wolf JM, Clauw DJ. Functional magnetic resonance imaging evidence of augmented pain processing in fibromyalgia. Arthritis Rheum 2002; 46: 1333-43.
27. Giesecke T, Williams DA, Harris RE, Cupps TR, Tian X, Tian TX, Gracely RH, Clauw DJ. Subgrouping of fibromyalgia patients on the basis of pressure-pain threshold and psychological factors. Arthritis Rheum 2003; 48: 2916-22.
28. Jensen KB, Kosek E, Petzke F, Carville S, Fransson P, Marcus H, Williams SC, Choy E, Giesecke T, Mainguy Y, Gracely R, Ingvar M. Evidence of dysfunctional pain inhibition in Fibromyalgia reflected in rACC during provoked pain. Pain 2009; 144: 95-100.
29. Jones AK, Brown WD, Friston KJ, Qi LY, Frackowiak RS. Cortical and subcortical localization of response to pain in man using positron emission tomography. Proc Biol Sci 1991; 244: 39-44.
30. Jones DK, Williams SC, Gasston D, Horsfield MA, Simmons A, Howard R. Isotropic resolution diffusion tensor imaging with whole brain acquisition in a clinically acceptable time. Hum Brain Mapp 2002; 15: 216-30.
31. Kim SG. Quantification of relative cerebral blood flow change by flow-sensitive alternating inversion recovery (FAIR) technique: application to functional mapping. Magn Reson Med 1995; 34: 293-301.
32. Kwiatek R, Barnden L, Tedman R, Jarrett R, Chew J, Rowe C, Pile K. Regional cerebral blood flow in fibromyalgia: single-photon-emission computed tomography evidence of reduction in the pontine tegmentum and thalami. Arthritis Rheum 2000; 43: 2823-33.
33. Kwong KK, Chesler DA, Weisskoff RM, Donahue KM, Davis TL, Ostergaard L, Campbell TA, Rosen BR. MR perfusion studies with T1-weighted echo planar imaging. Magn Reson Med 1995; 34: 878-87.
34. Law M. MR spectroscopy of brain tumors. Magn Reson Imaging 2004; 15:291-313.
35. Lee AD, Leow AD, Lu A, Reiss AL, Hall S, Chiang MC, Toga AW, Thompson, PM:. 3D pattern of brain abnormalities in Fragile X syndrome visualized using tensor-based morphometry. Neuroimage 2007; 34: 924–938.
36. Lentner C. (ed.). Geigy Scientific Tables, Vol. 4, p. 211, Ciba-Geigy Ltd, Basel, 1986.
37. Lepore, N, Brun C, Chou YY, Chiang MC, Dutton R, Hayashi K, Luders E, Lopez O, Aizenstein H, Toga A, Becker J, Thompson P: Generalized Tensor-Based Morphometry of HIV/AIDS Using Multivariate Statistics on Deformation Tensors. IEEE Transactions on Medical Imaging 2008; 27: 129–141.
38. Liu HL, Pu Y, Liu Y, Nickerson L, Andrews T, Fox PT, Gao JH. Cerebral blood flow measurement by dynamic contrast MRI using singular value decomposition with an adaptive threshold. Magn Reson Med 1999; 42:167-72.
39. Lutz J, Jager L, de Quervain D, Krauseneck T, Padberg F, Wichnalek M et al. White and gray matter abnormalities in the brain of patients with fibromyalgia: a diffusion-tensor and volumetric imaging study. Arthritis Rheum 2008; 58: 3960-9.
40. Maheshwari SR, Fatterpekar GM, Castillo M, Mukherji SK. Proton MR spectroscopy of the brain. Semin Ultrasound CT MR. 2000; 21: 434-51.

41. Mattson MP, Murrain M, Guthrie PB, and Kater SB. Fibroblast growth factor and glutamate: opposing roles in the generation and degeneration of hippocampal neuroarchitecture. J. Neurosci 1989; 9: 3728-3740.
42. Ostergaard L, Sorensen AG, Kwong KK, Weisskoff RM, Gyldensted C, Rosen BR. High resolution measurement of cerebral blood flow using intravascular tracer bolus passages. Part II: Experimental comparison and preliminary results. Magn Reson Med 1996; 36:726-36.
43. Petzke F, Clauw DJ, Ambrose K, Khine A, Gracely RH. Increased pain sensitivity in fibromyalgia: effects of stimulus type and mode of presentation. Pain 2003; 105: 403-13.
44. Provencher SW. Estimation of metabolite concentrations from localized in vivo proton NMR spectra. Magn Reson Med 1993; 30:672-9.
45. Purcell EU, Torrey HC, Pound RV. Resonance absorption by nuclear magnetic moments in a solid. Phys Rev 1946, 69:37-38.
46. Rajkowska G, Miguel-Hidalgo JJ. Gliogenesis and glial pathology in depression. CNS Neurol Disord Drug Targets 2007; 6: 219-33.
47. Rosen BR, Belliveau JW, Vevea JM, Brady TJ. Perfusion imaging with NMR contrast agents. Magn Reson Med 1990; 14: 249-65.
48. Sauter R, Schneider K, Wicklow K, Kolem H. Localized1H MRS of the human brain: Single-voxel versus CSI techniques. J. Magn Reson Imaging 1991, 1:241.
49. Silverstone PH, McGrath BM, Kim H. Bipolar disorder and myo-inositol: a review of the magnetic resonance spectroscopy findings. Bipolar Disord 2005; 7: 1-10.
50. Sundgren PC, Dong Q, Gómez-Hassan D, Mukherji SK, Maly P, Welsh R. Diffusion tensor imaging of the brain: review of clinical applications. Neuroradiology 2004; 46: 339-50.
51. Sundgren PC, Petrou M, Harris RE, Fan X, Foerster B, Mehrotra N et al. Diffusion-weighted and diffusion tensor imaging in fibromyalgia patients: a prospective study of whole brain diffusivity, apparent diffusion coefficient, and fraction anisotropy in different regions of the brain and correlation with symptom severity. Acad Radiol 2007; 14: 839-46.
52. Valet M, Gündel H, Sprenger T, Sorg C, Mühlau M, Zimmer C, Henningsen P, Tölle TR. Patients with pain disorder show gray-matter loss in pain-processing structures: a voxel-based morphometric study. Psychosom Med 2009; 71: 49-56.
53. Wolfe F, Smythe HA, Yunus MB, Bennet RM, Bombardier C, Goldenberg DL, Tugwell P, Campbell SM. The American College f Rheumatology 1990 Criteria for the classification of fibromyalgia. Report of the Multicenter Criteria Committee. Arthritis Rheum 1990; 33: 160-172.
54. Wolfe F, Ross K, Anderson J, Russell IJ. The prevalence and characteristics of fibromyalgia in the general population. Arthritis Rheum 1995; 38: 19-28.
55. Wolfe F. Fibromyalgia, the clinical syndrome. Rheum Dis Clin NA 1989; 15: 1-18.
56. Wolfe F, Anderson J, Harkness D, Bennet RM, Caro XJ, Goldenberg DL, Russell IJ, Wood PB, Ledbetter CR, Glabus MF, Broadwell LK, Patterson JC. Hippocampal metabolite abnormalities in fibromyalgia: correlation with clinical features. J Pain 2009; 10: 47-52.
57. Yildiz-Yesiloglu A, Ankerst DP. Neurochemical alterations of the brain in bipolar disorder and their implications for pathophysiology: a systematic review of the in vivo proton magnetic resonance spectroscopy findings. Prog Neuropsychopharmacol Biol Psychiatry 2006; 30: 969-95.

58. Yunus MB. Health status and disease severity in fibromyalgia: results of a six-center longitudinal study. Arthritis Rheum 1997; 40: 1571-79.

11. Annex. Some examples of new neuroimagen techniques in fibromyalgia.

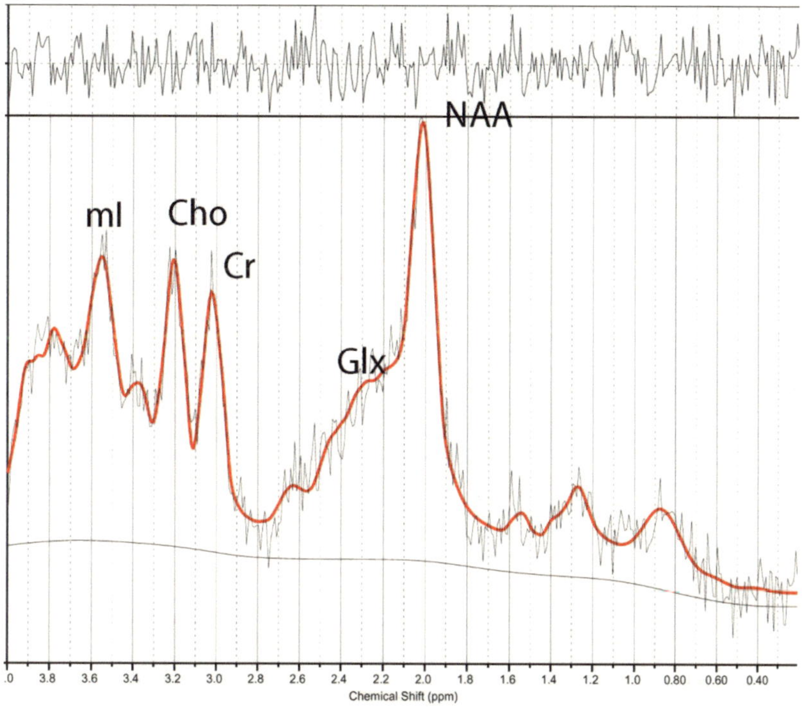

Fig. 1. Magnetic Resonance Spectroscopy

Typical in-vivo proton magnetic resonance spectrum depicts the localization of major peaks for *N*-acetylaspartate (2.02 ppm), creatine/phosphocreatine complex (3.02 ppm), choline (3.22 ppm), glutamine and glutamate (2.1 to 2.55 ppm); and myo-inositol (3.56 ppm)

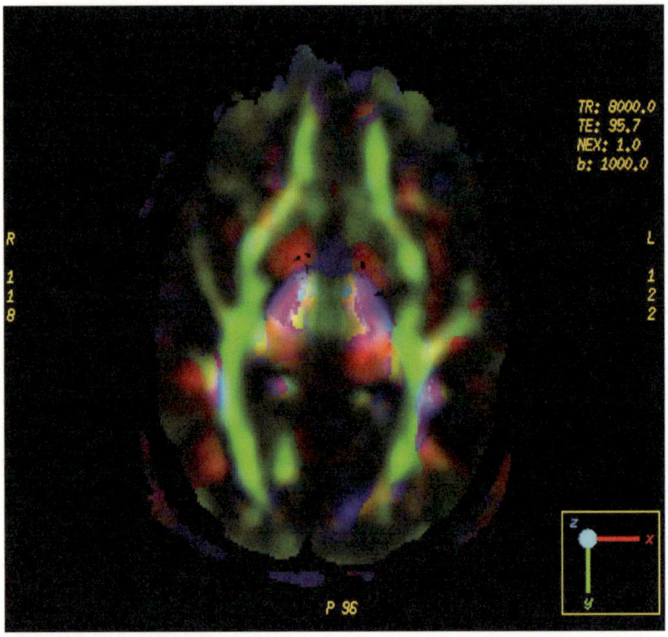

Fig. 2. Diffusion Tensor Imaging

Example of color-encoded fiber orientation maps. Fibers that are predominantly oriented left-right are shown in red, anterior-posterior fibers are shown in green, and superior-inferior fibers are shown in blue.

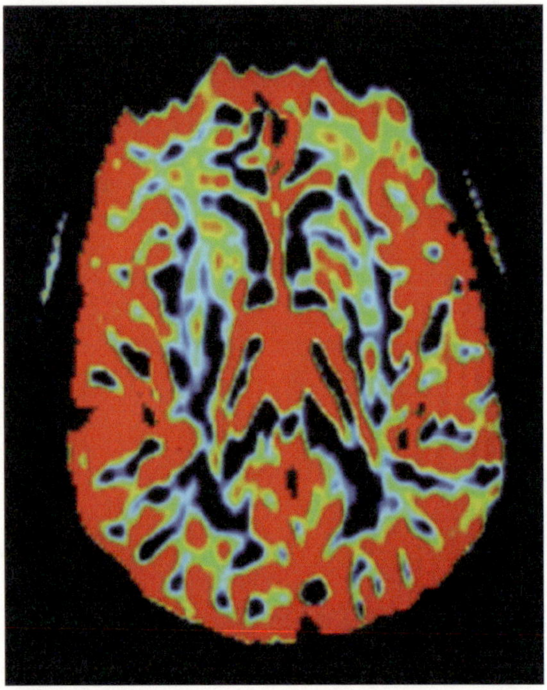

Fig. 3. Perfusion study

7

Restorative and compensatory changes in the brain during early motor recovery from hemiparetic stroke: a functional MRI study

Hiroyuki Kato[a] and Masahiro Izumiyama[b]
[a] *Department of Neurology, International University of Health and Welfare Hospital, Nasushiobara, Japan*
[b] *Department of Neurology, Sendai Nakae Hospital, Sendai, Japan*

1. Introduction

Stroke is a leading cause of disability in the elderly, and a considerable number of stroke patients suffer from residual motor deficits, particularly hemiparesis. There is a wide range of motor functional recovery after stroke, depending on the site, size and nature of the brain lesion (Duncan et al., 1992). Full recovery of hemiparesis is often observed when it is mild, and considerable recovery is not exceptional even after initial severe deficit. Functional recovery after stroke may be caused by resolution of acute effects of stroke, such as low blood flow, diaschisis and brain edema. However, functional gains may be prolonged past the period of this acute tissue response and its resolution. Stroke rehabilitation is introduced in order to promote brain plasticity and facilitate motor recovery. Understanding the mechanism of motor functional recovery after stroke is important because it may provide scientific basis for rehabilitation strategies.

Recent advances in non-invasive functional neuroimaging techniques, such as positron emission tomography (PET), functional MRI (fMRI) and near-infrared spectroscopy (NIRS), have enabled us to study directly the brain activity in humans after stroke (Herholz & Heiss, 2000; Calautti & Baron 2003; Rossini et al., 2003; Obrig & Villringer, 2003). Initial cross-sectional studies at chronic stages of stroke have demonstrated that the pattern of brain activation is different between paretic and normal hand movements, and suggested that long-term recovery is facilitated by compensation, recruitment and reorganization of cortical motor function in both damaged and non-damaged hemispheres (Chollet et al., 1991; Weiller et al., 1992; Cramer et al., 1997; Cao et al., 1998; Ward et al., 2003a). Subsequent longitudinal studies from subacute to chronic stages (before and after rehabilitation) have revealed a dynamic, bihemispheric reorganization of motor network, and emphasized the necessity of successive studies (Marshall et al., 2000; Calautti et al., 2001; Feydy et al., 2002; Ward et al, 2003b).

However, only limited data are available relating poststroke motor recovery to dynamic changes in cerebral cortical reorganization at the acute stage of stroke. We therefore measured the changes in cortical activation using fMRI during paretic hand movement both at the acute stage of stroke (the first study within 7 days of onset) and at the chronic stage when motor recovery was obtained.

2. Materials and Methods

2.1 Subjects

We selected 9 ischemic stroke patients with mild hemiparesis without a history of prior stroke, who received fMRI study within 7 days of stroke onset. The patients presented with neurological deficit including hemiparesis, and were admitted to our hospital. They received standard stroke therapy and rehabilitation, and were discharged from the hospital, when they were independent regarding activities of daily living. They were 58-85 years of age, 8 males and 1 female, and all of them were right-handed. All the cerebral infarcts were evidenced by MRI, and were located in various regions of the cerebrum. The hand motor area was preserved in all patients. Six of the patients had left hemiparesis and 3 had right hemiparesis. They could move their hands, even though weakly, when the first fMRI was performed. No patients in this study had language or attention deficits. Clinical data are summarized in Table 1. Nine right-handed, normal subjects (40-81 years of age; 3 males and 6 females) served as controls. This study was approved by the ethics committee of our hospital and informed consent was obtained from all subjects in accordance with the Declaration of Helsinki.

	Age Sex	H	Stroke location	PMH	first fMRI			second fMRI		
					day	GS	fMRI pattern	day	GS	fMRI pattern
1	76M	L	R MCA branches	af	1d	33/25	Red/ Add	29d	36/34	Red (Am)
2	83M	L	R MCA posterior branch	HT	3d	32/30	Red	35d	30/31	Norm
3	65M	L	R MCA	HT	4d	24/24	Red/ Add	28d	NA	Add
4	58M	L	R thalamus	HT DM	2d	32/27	Red/ Add	24d	35/33	Norm
5	85M	L	R corona radiata	HT DM	4d	12/0	Red	88d	17/8	Red (Am)
6	75F	L	R corona radiata	HT	7d	13/0	Add	48d	16/13	Norm
7	70M	R	L corona radiata	HT	5d	30/35	Red	26d	39/38	Norm
8	79M	R	L corona radiata	-	6d	29/31	Add	20d	25/30	Norm
9	78M	R	L MCA-PCA watershed	HT	7d	33/36	Red/ Add	31d	33/35	Norm

Table 1. Patient characteristics

M = male; F = female; H = hemiparesis; R = right; L = left; MCA = middle cerebral artery; PCA = posterior cerebral artery; PMH = past medical history; af = atrial fibrillation; HT = hypertension; DM = diabetes mellitus; GS = grip strength in kg for right hand/left hand; d = day; NA = not available; fMRI pattern, Red = reduced activation; Add = additional activation; Red(Am) = reduction ameliorated; Red/Add = reduced activation + additional activation; Norm = activation normalized

2.2 Functional MRI

Two fMRI studies were performed over time in all patients, the first one within 7 days of stroke onset (4.3 ± 2.1 days; the mean value ± SD) and the second one approximately 1 month later before they were discharged from the hospital (36.6 ± 20.9 days). The fMRI studies were performed using a 1.5 T Siemens Magnetom Symphony MRI scanner as described previously (Kato et al., 2002). Briefly, blood oxygenation level-dependent (BOLD) images (Ogawa et al., 1990) were obtained continuously in a transverse orientation using a gradient-echo, single shot echo planar imaging pulse sequence. The acquisition parameters were as follows: repetition time 3 s, time of echo 50 ms, flip angle 90°, 3-mm slice thickness, 30 slices through the entire brain, field of view 192 x 192 mm, and 128 x 128 matrix.

During the fMRI scan, the patients and normal controls performed sequential, self-paced hand movements (repeated closing and opening of the hand). This task performance occurred in periods of 30 s, interspaced with 30 s rest periods. The cycle of rest and task was repeated 5 times during each hand movement. Therefore, the fMRI scan of each hand movement took 5 min to complete, producing 3,000 images. A staff member monitored the patient directly throughout the study, and gave the start and stop signals by tapping gently on the knee, and confirmed the absence of mirror movements. All the stroke patients completed the task but the paretic hand movement appeared abnormal at the acute stage.

Data analysis was performed using Statistical Parametric Mapping (SPM) 99 (Wellcome Department of Cognitive Neurology, London, UK, http://www.fil.ion.ucl.ac.uk/spm/) implemented in MATLAB (The MathWorks Inc., Natick, MA, USA). After realignment and smoothing, the general linear model was employed for the detection of activated voxels. The voxels were considered as significantly activated if $p<0.05$ (corrected for multiple comparison). All the measurements were performed with this same statistical threshold. The activation images were overlaid on corresponding T1-weighted anatomic images.

The criteria for the changes in the fMRI activation pattern in stroke patients were as follows. 1. A reduction of activation was considered when the area of activation was reduced to <50% compared to that induced by unaffected hand movement of the patient. 2. An expansion of activation was considered when the area of activation was increased by >50% compared with that induced by unaffected hand movement. 3. An appearance of activation was considered when a cluster of activation was induced in a region where unaffected hand movement induced no or little activation.

3. Results

3.1 Control subjects

In control subjects, each hand movement activated predominantly the contralateral primary sensorimotor cortex (SM1), supplementary motor areas (SMA), and the ipsilateral anterior lobe of the cerebellum (Cbll) (Fig. 1). Contralateral SM1 and ipsilateral Cbll were always involved with a variation between individuals, and SMA was activated in 6 of 9 subjects with more variation. Ipsilateral SM1 was slightly activated in 2 of 9 control subjects. There was no large difference between right and left hand movements.

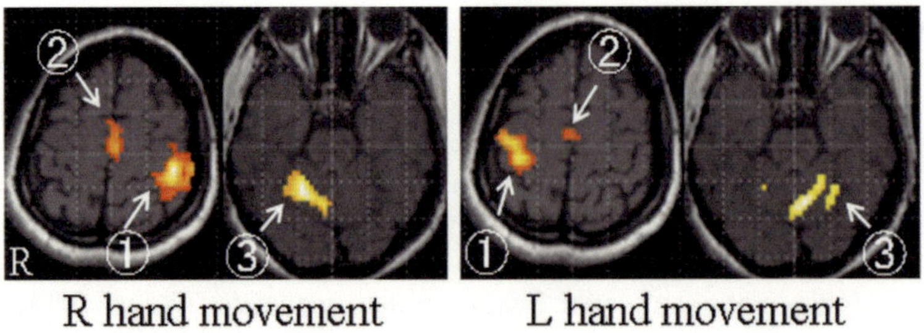

Fig.1. fMRI of a 40-year old normal female. Right or left hand movement activated contralateral primary sensorimotor cortex (①), supplementary motor areas (②), and ipsilateral anterior lobe of the cerebellum (③). There was no large difference between activations during right and left hand movements.

3.2 Stroke patients

During unaffected hand movements, the patients activated the same motor cortical areas as the control subjects did.

The brain activation pattern during paretic hand movements within 7 days of stroke onset (the first fMRI) was different from that during unaffected or normal hand movements (Figs. 2-4). There were two major findings.

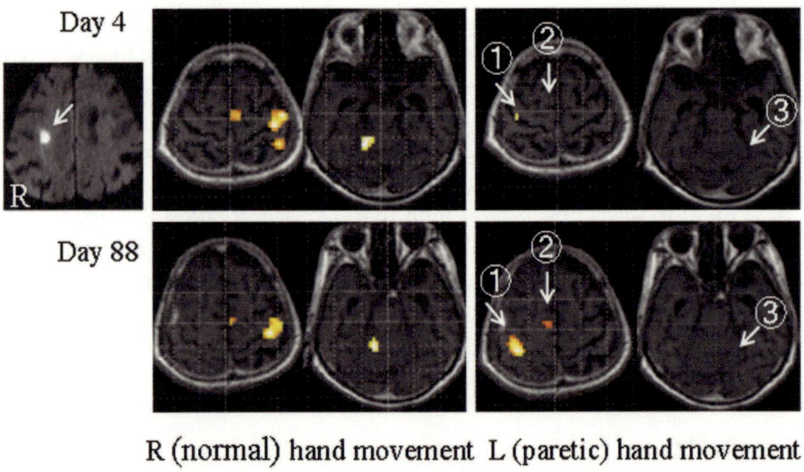

Fig. 2. fMRI of a 85-year old man (patient 5) who had a cerebral infarct in the right corona radiata near the motor hand area (arrow on the diffusion-weighted MRI). After 4 days of stroke onset, right (normal) hand movement induced a normal activation pattern in the left primary sensorimotor cortex, supplementary motor areas, and right cerebellum. During left (paretic) hand movement, activation in contralateral primary sensorimotor cortex (①) was reduced and no activation was seen in the supplementary motor areas (②) and the cerebellum (③). After 88 days, both right (normal) and left (paretic) hand movements induced a normal activation pattern except that no activation was induced in the cerebellum (③) during left (paretic) hand movement.

First, activations were reduced or lost in part or all of the normally activated regions (contralateral SM1, SMA, and ipsilateral Cbll) in 8 of 9 patients. Activation in contralateral SM1 was reduced or lost in 5 of 9 patients; in 4 of 4 patients with cortical infarction (Fig. 3) and in 1 of 5 patients with subcortical infarction (Fig. 2). In the latter patient, subcortical infarct was located near the motor hand area. In 4 of 5 patients with subcortical infarction, in contrast, activation in contralateral SM1 was preserved. Even when contralateral SM1 was activated, there was a posterior or ventral shift or expansion of activation in 2 patients.
Ipsilateral cerebellar activation was reduced or lost in 5 of 9 patients. SMA activation was reduced or lost in 4 of 7 patients who activated SMA during unaffected hand movement.
Second, a recruitment of additional motor-related areas was seen in 4 of 9 patients. The additional activations were observed in ipsilateral SM1 (4 patients), contralateral Cbll (1 patient), premotor cortex (bilateral in 1 patient and ipsilateral in 1 patient), and bilateral parietal cortex (1 patient) (Fig. 4).
At the second fMRI study approximately 1 month later, the brain activation pattern during paretic hand movement had returned to normal in 7 of 9 patients and near normal in 2 other patients. Additional activation was still seen in ipsilateral SM1 in 1 patient.

4. Discussion

In this study, we observed a remarkable difference in cerebral cortical activation between affected and unaffected hand movements at the acute stage of stroke (within 7 days of onset). Paretic hand movement-induced brain activation may be reduced markedly in cortical areas that are normally activated by unaffected hand movements (contralateral SM1, SMA, and ipsilateral Cbll). The reduction of SM1 activation was observed predominantly in patients with cortical infarction and was exceptional in patients with subcortical infarction. Early recruitment of additional motor-related areas (ipsilateral SM1 in particular and secondary motor areas) may occur. At the chronic stage (the second fMRI), brain activations during paretic hand movement had returned to normal or near-normal. Thus, early motor recovery after stroke was accompanied by two major changes on fMRI, i.e., restoration of brain activity and recruitment of additional brain activity.
We wanted to investigate into motor-related brain activation, and selected such patients who could move their hands, even though weakly, when the first fMRI study was performed within 7 days of stroke onset. As a result, we needed to select stroke patients with mild motor deficit and resultant excellent recovery because patients with poor motor function cannot perform the task of this study. This a priori limited the scope of the findings of our study. Furthermore, the motor performance of the paretic hand was not normal and one may point out that the brain activities during paretic and unaffected hand movements cannot be compared.
But our results suggest that motor functional recovery occurred primarily using the standard motor system when damage to it was mild or partial, recruiting functionally related motor areas when necessary as a compensatory strategy. The recruitment of additional activation of motor-related areas was often transient. Therefore, this additional activation may reflect compensation and unmasking or disinhibition of existing motor network which is masked or inhibited under normal conditions since the activation appeared early after stroke. Of interest is that these restorative and compensatory changes occurred within the first month after stroke, and this period seemed critical to motor functional recovery.

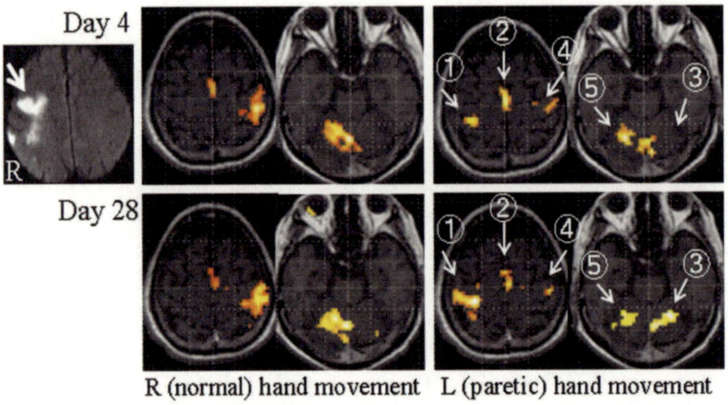

Fig. 3. fMRI of a 65-year old man (patient 3) who had a cerebral infarct in the right middle cerebral artery territory (arrow on the diffusion-weighted MRI). After 4 days of stroke onset, right (normal) hand movement induced normal activation in the left primary sensorimotor cortex, supplementary motor areas, and the right cerebellum. During left (paretic) hand movement, activation in the contralateral primary sensorimotor cortex (①) was reduced and that in the ipsilateral cerebellum (③) was lost. Activations in ipsilateral primary motor cortex (④) and contralateral cerebellum (⑤) were observed. Activation in the supplementary motor areas (②) appeared normal. After 28 days, activations in contralateral primary sensorimotor cortex (①) and ipsilateral cerebellum (③) had been normalized. Activations in ipsilateral primary motor cortex (④) and contralateral cerebellum (⑤) were still seen. Right (normal) hand movement induced a normal activation pattern.

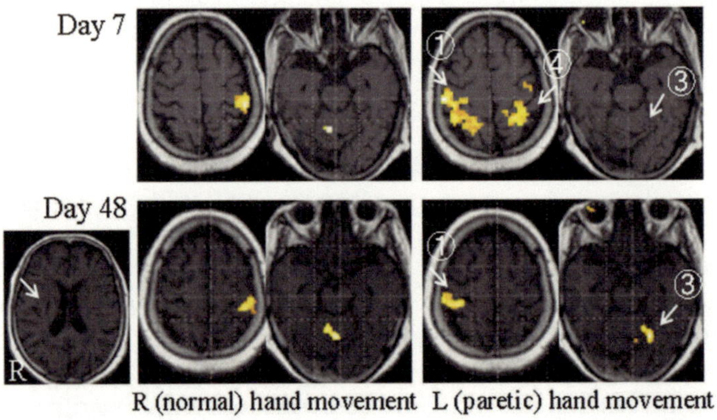

Fig. 4. fMRI of a 75-year old female (patient 6) who had a cerebral infarct in the right corona radiata (arrow on the T1-weighted MRI). After 7 days of stroke onset, right (normal) hand movement induced normal activation in the left primary sensorimotor cortex and the right cerebellum. No activation was seen in the supplementary motor areas in this patient. During left (paretic) hand movement, extensive activation was seen in bilateral primary sensorimotor and parietal cortices (① and ④) but no activation was seen in the supplementary motor areas and the cerebellum (③). After 48 days, both paretic (left) and normal (right) hand movements induced a normal activation pattern.

Earlier functional neuroimaging studies on poststroke cerebral reorganization from subacute to chronic stages revealed several activation patterns during paretic hand movement (Ward & Cohen, 2004; Jang, 2007). These include (1) a posterior shift of contralateral SM1 activation (Pineiro et al., 2001; Calautti et al., 2003) or peri-infarct reorganization after primary motor cortex infarction (Cramer et al., 1997; Jang et al., 2005a), (2) a shift of primary motor cortex activation to the ipsilateral (contralesional) cortex (Chollet et al., 1991; Marshall et al., 2000; Feydy et al., 2002), (3) contribution of the secondary motor areas (Cramer et al., 1997; Carey et al., 2002; Ward et al., 2006), and (4) higher contralateral activity in the cerebellar hemisphere (Small et al., 2002). In the present study, we observed similar additional activation patterns at the acute stage of stroke. The earlier studies have also shown that the expanded activations may later decrease with functional improvements, which was also true in many of our acute stroke patients. The contralesional shift of activation may return to ipsilesional SM1 activation with functional gains (Feydy et al., 2002; Takeda et al., 2007), but worse outcome may correlate with a shift in the balance of activation toward the contralesional SM1 (Calautti et al., 2001; Feydy et al., 2002; Zemke et al., 2003). Thus, the patterns of cerebral activation evoked by hand movement show impaired organization and reorganization of brain motor network, and best recovery may depend on how much original motor system is reusable. The patterns of activation may also be dependent on the patient's ability to recruit residual portions of the bilateral motor network (Silvestrini et al., 1998).

The fMRI findings need to be considered within the context of technical and task-dependent factors. The fMRI mapping obtained by the BOLD technique is dependent on the spatial extent of hemodynamic changes induced by local synaptic activity and field potentials (Logothetis et al., 2001). Localization of neural activity may be confounded by many factors (Ugurbil et al., 2003). BOLD-dependent capillary density and draining veins and the perfusion of brain tissue may differ between damaged and undamaged tissues, especially at acute stages of stroke. fMRI activation can even be lost in stroke patients because of altered vasomotor reactivity, demonstrating uncoupling of neuronal activity and fMRI activation (Rossini et al., 2004; Binkofski & Seitz 2004; Murata et al., 2006). In our study, paretic hand movement at the acute stage resulted in reduced motor cortex activation in the damaged hemisphere, especially in patients with cortical infarction. This reduced activation may be due not only to impaired neural activity but also to this uncoupling when cerebral infarction was close to the SM1. Thus, we need to be cautious when interpreting fMRI results at the acute stage of stroke. In contrast, patients with subcortical infarction did not usually display a reduction in motor cortex activation because the lesion was distant from the motor cortex.

Of interest is the determinant of fMRI activation patterns induced by paretic hand movement. Motor system reorganization may also be influenced by stroke topography (Feydy et al., 2002; Luft et al., 2004), time after stroke (Ward et al., 2004), and stroke side (Zemke et al., 2003). Cortical motor organizations between dominant and non-dominant hand movements may be different, and non-dominant hand movements are more bilaterally organized (Kim et al., 1993). Furthermore, the performance of complex motor tasks is accompanied by bilateral activation of motor cortices in contrast to simple motor tasks that result in only contralateral activation (Shibasaki et al., 1993). Hemiparesis would increase task difficulty. When task demand increases, more regions would be activated by a motor task. Improvement in motor skills may depend on rehabilitation, handedness, motivation, and age-related capacity for plasticity. Then motor reorganization after stroke may be obtained depending on a number of factors. If motor reorganization is related to the degree of damage to the pyramidal tract, information on the sensorimotor projections would help further understand the brain reorganization in the context of structure and function. Diffusion tensor imaging tractography, which non-invasively visualize the pyramidal tract using the water molecule diffusion characteristics in the white matter, may be the tool to analyze its integrity (Masutani et al., 2003). The combination of fMRI and tractography of the pyramidal tract would further elucidate the mechanism of motor functional recovery after stroke (Jang et al., 2005b).

The ipsilateral primary motor cortex activation may be seen slightly in normal subjects and we cannot distinguish whether the ipsilateral motor activities found in stroke patients existed prior to stroke or are a result of brain plasticity. Furthermore, we do not know whether additional activation that appeared after stroke really contributed to motor functional recovery. With regard to these fundamental points, of interest are the findings of experimental studies using animal models. Nishimura et al. (2007) have shown using a monkey model of unilateral pyramidal tract injury that motor recovery involves bilateral primary motor cortex during the early recovery stage and more extensive regions of contralesional primary motor cortex and bilateral premotor cortex during the late recovery stage. Nudo et al. (1996) and Frost et al. (2003) used an ischemic brain injury model in the monkey and showed substantial enlargement of the hand representation within the primary motor cortex and the ventral premotor cortex. These animal studies suggest that reorganization in brain motor network provides a neural substrate for adaptive motor behavior and plays a critical role in the recovery of motor function after stroke.

5. Conclusion

We investigated the changes in cortical activation using fMRI during paretic hand movement both at the acute stage of stroke and at the chronic stage when motor recovery was obtained. The findings of this study suggest that early motor recovery after stroke occurs primarily using the standard motor system, by recovering from reversible injury and by recruiting related motor areas for functional compensation. fMRI is an important tool for revealing the capacity and progress of rehabilitation-dependent changes in the brain motor network after stroke, and provides a neuroscientific basis for stroke rehabilitation. Future studies should clarify the relation between the motor recovery mechanisms and clinical outcome, and the importance of the critical period that greatly influences motor functional recovery after stroke.

6. Acknowledgments

We thank the staff members of the MRI section of Sendai Nakae Hospital, Ms. Fumi Kozuka, Ms. Satsuki Ohi, Mr. Takeru Ohmukai, Ms. Yoko Sato, Ms. Aya Kanai, and Mr. Katsuhiro Aki, for their help to perform fMRI studies. We also thank Dr. Naohiro Saito, Department of Physiology, Tohoku University School of Medicine, Sendai, Japan, for his expert assistance on the fMRI-spm99 analysis.

This study was supported by Grant-in-Aid for Scientific Research (16500352 and 19500458), Japan Society for the Promotion of Science, and by CREST, Japan Science and Technology Agency.

7. References

Binkofski, F. & Seitz, R.J. (2004). Modulation of the BOLD-response in early recovery from sensorimotor stroke. *Neurology,* 63, 1223-1229

Calautti, C.; Leroy, F.; Guincestre, J.Y. & Baron, J.-C. (2001). Dynamics of motor network overactivation after striatocapsular stroke: a longitudinal PET study using a fixed-performance paradigm. *Stroke,* 32, 2534-2542

Calautti, C. & Baron, J.-C. (2003). Functional neuroimaging studies of motor recovery after stroke in adults. A review. *Stroke,* 34, 1553-1566

Calautti, C.; Leroy, F.; Guincestre, J.Y. & Baron, J.-C. (2003). Displacement of primary sensorimotor cortex activation after subcortical stroke: a longitudinal PET study with clinical correlation. *Neuroimage,* 19, 1650-1654

Cao, Y.; D'Olhaberriague, L.; Vikingstad, E.M.; Levine, S.R. & Welch, K.M.A. (1998). Pilot study of functional MRI to assess cerebral activation of motor function after poststroke hemiparesis. *Stroke,* 29, 112-122

Carey, J.R.; Kimberley, T.J.; Lewis, S.M.; Auerbach, E.J.; Dorsey L.; Rundquist, P. & Ugurbil. K. (2002). Analysis of fMRI and finger tracking training in subjects with chronic stroke. *Brain,* 125, 773-788

Chollet, F.; DiPiero, V.; Wise, R.J.S.; Brooks, D.J.; Dolan, R.J. & Fracowiak, R.S.J. (1991). The functional anatomy of motor recovery after stroke in humans: a study with positron emission tomography. *Ann. Neurol.,* 29, 63-71

Cramer, S.C.; Nelles, G.; Benson, R.R.; Kaplan, J.D.; Parker, R.A.; Kwong, K.K.; Kennedy, D.N.; Finklestein, S.P. & Rosen, B.R. (1997). A functional MRI study of subjects recovered from hemiparetic stroke. *Stroke,* 28, 2518-2527

Duncan, P.W.; Goldstein, L.B.; Matchar, D.; Divine, G.W. & Feussner, J. (1992). Measurement of motor recovery after stroke: outcome measures and sample size requirements. *Stroke,* 23, 1084-1089

Feydy, A.; Carlier, R.; Rody-Brami, A.; Bussel, B.; Cazalis, F.; Pierot, L.; Burnod, Y. & Maier, M.A. (2002). Longitudinal study of motor recovery after stroke: recruitment and focusing of brain activation. *Stroke,* 33, 1610-1617

Frost, S.B.; Barbay, S.; Friel, K.M.; Plautz, E.J. & Nudo, R.J. (2003). Reorganization of remote cortical regions after ischemic brain injury: a potential substrate for stroke recovery. *J. Neurophysiol.,* 89, 3205-3214

Herholz, A. & Heiss, W.-D. (2000). Functional imaging correlates of recovery after stroke in humans. *J. Cereb. Blood Flow Metab.,* 20, 1619-1631

Jang S.H. (2007). A review of motor recovery mechanisms in patients with stroke. *NeuroRehabilitation,* 22, 253-259

Jang, S.H.; Ahn, S.H.; Yang, D.S.; Lee, D.K.; Kim, D.K. & Son, S.M. (2005a). Cortical reorganization of hand motor function to primary sensory cortex in hemiparetic patients with a primary motor cortex infarct. *Arch. Phys. Med. Rehabil.,* 86, 1706-1708

Jang, S.H.; Kwon, Y.-H.; You, S.H.; Song, J.C.; Lee, M.Y.; Kim, J.H.; Park, K.H. & Cho, Y.W. (2005b). Medial reorganization of motor function demonstrated by functional MRI and diffusion tensor tractography. *Restor. Neurol. Neurosci.,* 23, 265-269

Kato, H.; Izumiyama, M.; Koizumi, H.; Takahashi, A. & Itoyama, Y. (2002). Near-infrared spectroscopic topography as a tool to monitor motor reorganization after hemiparetic stroke. A comparison with functional MRI. *Stroke,* 33, 2032-2036

Kim, S.-G.; Ashe, J.; Hendrich, K.; Ellermann, J.M.; Merkle, H.; Ugurbil, K. & Georgopoulos, A.P. (1993). Functional magnetic resonance imaging of motor cortex: hemispheric asymmetry and handedness. *Science,* 261, 615-617

Logothetis, N.; Pauls, J.; Augath, M.; Trinath, T. & Oeltermann, A. (2001). Neurophysiological investigation of the basis of the fMRI signal. *Nature,* 412, 150-157

Luft, A.R.; Waller, S.; Forrester, L.; Smith, G.V.; Whitall, J.; Macko, R.F.; Schulz, J.B. & Hanley, D.F. (2004). Lesion location alters brain activation in chronically impaired stroke survivors. *Neuroimage,* 21, 924-935

Marshall, R.S.; Perera, G.M.; Lazar, R.M.; Krakauer, J.W.; Constantine, R.C. & DeLaPaz, R.L. (2000). Evolution of cortical activation during recovery from corticospinal tract infarction. *Stroke,* 31, 656-661

Masutani, Y.; Aoki, S.; Abe, O.; Hayashi, N. & Otomo, K. (2003). MR diffusion tensor imaging: recent advance and new techniques for diffusion tensor visualization. *Eur. J. Radiol.,* 46, 53-66

Murata, Y.; Sakatani, K.; Hoshino, T.; Fujiwara, N.; Kano, T.; Nakamura, S. & Katayama, Y. (2006). Effects of cerebral ischemia on evoked cerebral blood oxygenation responses and BOLD contrast functional MRI in stroke patients. *Stroke,* 37, 2514-2520

Nishimura, Y.; Onoe, H.; Morichika, Y.; Perfiliev, S.; Tsukada, H. & Isa, T. (2007). Time-dependent central compensatory mechanisms of finger dexterity after spinal cord injury. *Science,* 318, 1150-1155

Nudo, R.J.; Wise, B.M.; SiFuentes, F. & Milliken, G.W. (1996). Neural substrate for the effects of rehabilitative training on motor recovery after ischemic infarct. *Science,* 272, 1791-1794

Obrig, H. & Villringer, A. (2003). Beyond the visible – imaging the human brain with light. *J. Cereb. Blood Flow Metab.,* 23, 1-18

Ogawa, S.; Lee, T.M.; Kay, A.R. & Tank, D.W. (1990). Brain magnetic resonance imaging with contrast dependent on blood oxygenation. *Proc. Natl. Acad. Sci. U.S.A.,* 87, 9868-9872

Pineiro, R.; Pendlebury, S.; Johansen-Berg, H. & Matthews, P.M. (2001). Functional MRI detects posterior shifts in primary sensorimotor cortex activation after stroke. Evidence of local adaptive reorganization? *Stroke,* 32, 1134-1139

Rossini, P.M.; Calautti, C.; Pauri, F. & Baron, J.C. (2003). Post-stroke plastic reorganization in the adult brain. *Lancet Neurol.,* 2, 493-502

Rossini, P.M.; Altamura, C.; Ferretti, A.; Vernieri, F.; Zappasodi, F.; Caulo, M.; Pizzella, V.; Del Gratta, C.; Romani, G.-L. & Tecchio, F. (2004). Does cerebrovascular disease affect the coupling between neuronal activity and local haemodynamics? *Brain,* 127, 99-110

Shibasaki, H.; Sadato, N.; Lyshkow, H.; Yonekura, Y.; Honda, M.; Nagamine, T.; Suwazono, S.; Magata, Y.; Ikeda, A.; Miyazaki, M.; Fukuyama, H.; Asato, R. & Konishi, J. (1993). Both primary motor cortex and supplementary motor area play an important role in complex finger movement. *Brain,* 116, 1387-1398

Silvestrini, M.; Cupini, L.M.; Placidi, F.; Diomedi, M. & Bernardi, G. (1998). Bilateral hemispheric activation in the early recovery of motor function after stroke. *Stroke,* 29, 1305-1310

Small, A.L.; Hlustik, P.; Noll, D.C.; Genovese, C. & Solodkin, A. (2002) Cerebellar hemispheric activation ipsilateral to the paretic hand correlates with functional recovery after stroke. *Brain,* 125, 1544-1557

Takeda, K.; Gomi, Y.; Imai, I.; Shimoda, N.; Hiwatari, M. & Kato, H. (2007). Shift of motor activation areas during recovery from hemiparesis after cerebral infarction: a longitudinal study with near-infrared spectroscopy. *Neurosci. Res.*, 59, 136-144

Ugurbil, K.; Toth, L. & Kim, D.S. (2003). How accurate is magnetic resonance imaging of brain function? *Trends Neurosci.*, 26, 108-114

Ward, N.S.; Brown, M.M.; Thompson, A.J. & Frackowiak, R.S.J. (2003a). Neural correlates of outcome after stroke: a cross-sectional fMRI study. *Brain*, 126, 1430-1448

Ward, N.S.; Brown, M.M.; Thompson, A.J. & Frackowia, R.S.J. (2003b). Neural correlates of motor recovery after stroke: a longitudinal fMRI study. *Brain*, 126, 2476-2496

Ward, N.S.; Brown, M.M.; Thompson, A.J. & Frackowiak, R.S.J. (2004). The influence of time after stroke on brain activations during a motor task. *Ann. Neurol.*, 55, 829-834

Ward, N.S. & Cohen, L.G. (2004). Mechanisms underlying recovery of motor function after stroke. *Arch. Neurol.*, 61, 1844-1848

Ward, N.S.; Newton, J.M.; Swayne, O.B.; Lee, L.; Thompson, A.J.; Greenwood, R.J.; Rothwell, J.C. & Frackowiak, R.S. (2006). Motor system activation after subcortical stroke depends on corticospinal system integrity. *Brain*, 129(Pt. 3), 809-819

Weiller, C.; Chollet, F.; Friston, K.J.;Wise, R.J. & Frackowiak, R.S. (1992). Functional reorganization of the brain in recovery from striatocapsular infarction in man. *Ann. Neurol.*, 315, 463-472

Zemke, A.C.; Heagerty, P.J.; Lee, C. & Cramer, S.C. (2003). Motor cortex organization after stroke is related to side of stroke and level of recovery. *Stroke*, 34, e23-28